This book was written to b
inclusive of everything yo
could read Harrisons, upto
approaches to common wo.

This book is meant more for hospital based medicine rather than outpatient. However, a lot of the diseases and workups in the text are common/overlap to the outpatient setting, and include what a primary care physician should be doing to prevent disease in a patient and what to do post hospitalization.

The text starts with common workups. These may include things you are paged for about a patient you are taking care of or when cross covering, rapid responses, or new patients that are being admitted from the ED. It is a quick approach to the patient with their complaint, and things you should look out for and not miss. Management in this section is brief, but allows you to stabilize/support the patient while you come up with their diagnosis and ongoing treatment plan.

The next section is common diseases seen in the field of internal medicine. These chosen diseases are based on both personal experience and research. It is obviously not inclusive to all patients you will see in the hospital as the scope of that is too broad for this book. It is meant to cover the bread and butter of internal medicine. Each section includes the approach to the history/physical, differential, labs/imaging, diagnostic/treatment algorithms, treatment, etiologies, risk factors, pathogenesis, complications, prevention, and general admission orders. Included in this section are landmark clinical trials that support the information in the text.

There is a section on miscellaneous topics in internal medicine, such as inpatient diabetes management, approach to reading CXRs/EKGs, etc.

Not everyone will go on to become a pulmonary/critical care physician, but you may be spending a good amount of time in the ICU. I have placed a section specifically for ICU basics that every internal medicine professional should understand, such as DKA, shock differential, vasopressors, and indications for intubation. This section is obviously not inclusive of all you will need to know.

The last section is common drugs you will be prescribing.

My sources included Harrisons, Pocket Medicine, uptodate, MKSAP, etc. I tried to be as evidenced based as I could. Clinical trials are referenced throughout; however, other sources are not referenced as the information presented is available in many different forms. Please use this text as a guide, and any errors in this book were not intentional, as I am still learning this complex field of medicine that we all chose to be a part of.

I hope this helps in your journey through medicine.

Your friend,
Mitchell Edwards, D.O.

Mitchell Edwards, D.O.
Guide to the Most Common Internal Medicine Workups and Diseases
Copyright 2017
All rights reserved
ISBN 9781521544914
Independently Published

Sources and thanks, not limited to, Uptodate, Harrisons Principals to Internal Medicine 19th Edition, Pocket Medicine 5th Edition, MKSAP 17, and Online MedEd for the framework of material that may be included in this text.

The journey to create this text has been long. I started this book with hand written notes in a notebook I brought with me to rounds every day in my 3rd and 4th year clerkships in Internal Medicine. After I had many topics written, I decided to transcribe the often illegible notes into a word document. In this process, I made sure all facts written were based off evidence based medicine, or from well-respected sources (such as the ones above). From there, I added figures/algorithms (as you may be able to tell, these were made myself, with very little computer skills) to help organize the workups in the text. As I went on to my medicine residency, I added sections that I saw frequently in the hospital, and also added references to clinical trials supporting the information in the text. I have published this text at the end of my intern year, and will continue updating this for new editions as medicine is forever evolving.

Special thanks to the University of California Irvine Internal Medicine program, including the faculty, and my amazing resident colleagues. I could not have written this book without your expertise and tremendous support. It does not feel like work when I get to practice medicine with all of you.

And to my wife Nicole- your endless support throughout this crazy journey has been unmeasurable. Without you, nothing in my life would be what it is today. I love you with all of my heart. Thank you for being my best friend.

Table of Contents

Common Workups in Internal Medicine..5

Chest Pain..5

Abdominal Pain..7

Headache..9

Hypotension...11

Hypertension..13

Common Arrhythmias..14

Fever..16

Shortness of Breath..18

GI Bleeding..20

Common Diseases in Internal Medicine..22

Urinary Tract Infections...22

Pneumonia...29

COPD...37

Asthma...46

Pleural Effusion...55

Venous Thromboembolism (PE/DVT)..62

Acute Coronary Syndrome..73

Heart Failure..87

Atrial Fibrillation...102

Syncope..111

Upper/Lower GI Bleeding...121

Chronic Liver Disease/Cirrhosis Complications...............................131

Acute Pancreatitis..144

Acute Kidney Injury..152

Chronic Kidney Disease..162

Hyponatremia..171

Anemia..177

Thrombocytopenia...187

Transient Ischemic Attacks and Ischemic Stroke..............................194

Acute Confusion/Delirium...204

Approach to the Acutely Ill Infected Febrile Patient.........................211

Sepsis Spectrum...215

Infectious Endocarditis..230

Acute Bacterial/Aseptic Meningitis..238
Cellulitis..250
Osteomyelitis...254
Miscellaneous Topics in Internal Medicine..259
Inpatient Diabetes Management...259
Hemoptysis..260
Back Pain..260
Diarrhea..261
Alcohol Withdrawal...262
Approach to LFTs..263
Approach to Pain Control...264
Approach to Reading Chest X-Rays...266
Approach to Reading EKGs..268
Approach to Arterial Blood Gases...275
Electrolyte Repletion..277
Basic ICU Topics..279
Shock Differential...279
Vasopressors..281
Indications for Intubation and Ventilatory Weaning..281
DKA Initial Labs and Management..284
Common Medications..286
Cardiac Medications...286
Respiratory Medications..287
Gastrointestinal Medications...288
Antibiotics...289

Common Workups in Internal Medicine

Chest Pain

Differential:

- **Heart/vascular:**
    - Angina
    - MI
    - Acute pericarditis
    - Aortic dissection
- **Lungs:**
    - Pneumonia
    - PE
    - Pneumothorax
- **GI:**
    - GERD
    - Peptic ulcer disease
    - Pancreatitis
    - Diffuse esophageal spasm
- **Other:**
    - Costochondritis
    - Rib fracture
    - Anxiety
    - Herpes zoster
    - Skin lacerations
    - Muscle strain
- **Things you do not want to miss:**
    - MI
    - Aortic dissection
    - PE
    - Pneumothorax

Key History:

- **It may be myocardial ischemia or something else life threatening, so should see the patient ASAP**
- What are the patient's vitals?
- What was the patient admitted for?
- Where is the pain?
- Is it worsened with exertion and relieved by rest?
- Is it improved with nitroglycerin?
- Associated symptoms:
    - Presyncope?
    - SOB?
    - Diaphoresis?
- Risk factors for ACS/CAD:
    - Smoking
    - Diabetes
    - HTN
    - Dyslipidemia

- o Obesity
- How far can you walk without stopping? What stops you?
- Is the pain associated with your breathing (pleuritic)?
- Is it tender to touch?
- Does the pain occur when you move?
- What is the blood pressure on both arms (is it the same)?
- Quick chart review

Focused Examination:

- General: does the patient appear distressed or ill?
- Vitals:
    - o Hypotension is an omnious sign
    - o Tachycardia may be from a PE or from pain
    - o Bradycardia may be from AV block with inferior MI
    - o BP in both arms for aortic dissection evaluation
    - o Fever may raise suspicion for PE or pericarditis
- Chest:
    - o Chest wall tenderness, skin lesions
    - o Murmurs, rubs, gallops
    - o JVP
- Respiratory:
    - o Listen for crackles, absent breath sounds on one side
    - o Friction rub
- Abdomen:
    - o Examine for distension, tenderness, and bowel sounds
- Extremities:
    - o Edema or evidence of DVT
    - o Examine pulses bilaterally in both upper and lower extremities to assess for dissection

Labs/Diagnostics:

- EKG, review telemetry if available
- ABG if respiratory distress or low saturations are present
- Serial troponins
- CXR
- Consider CT angiogram or V/Q scan if PE suspected
- Consider contrast CT or TEE if aortic dissection is suspected

Management:

- **Initial orders:**
    - o Stat EKG with continuous monitoring, troponin
    - o O2 to keep O2 sats >92%
    - o Sublingual nitroglycerin 0.4 mg
    - o Aspirin 325 mg
    - o Confirm IV access
- If evidence of acute MI on EKG (ST elevation of 1 mm or more in two contiguous leads or new LBBB):
    - o Call stat cardiology consult for consideration of reperfusion therapy (thrombolytics or angioplasty)

- On telemetry monitoring, IV access, oxygen 2L NC
- Consider beta blockers, nitrates, morphine, heparin
- If chest pain persists, consider clopidogrel
- If aortic dissection:
    - Immediate transfer to CCU/MICU
    - Start nitroprusside and/or labetalol for BP control
    - Stat vascular/thoracic surgery consult
- If PE:
    - Supplemental O2
    - LMWH or UFH
- Pneumothorax:
    - Tension pneumothorax requires immediate needle decompression in 2nd intercostal space in midclavicular line, followed by chest tube
    - Other pneumothoraces involving >20% of lung require surgery consult for chest tube placement
- GI:
    - Antacids, famotidine, or omeprazole
    - Elevate head of bed, especially after meals
- Refractory chest pain:
    - Re-evaluate what you thought was the cause of the chest pain
    - Repeat EKG, vitals, physical exam
    - For ongoing cardiac ischemia with elevated troponins and/or ST segment depression, start a nitroglycerin drip, consider clopidogrel, and consider urgent cardiology consult

Abdominal Pain

Differential:

- **Things you do not want to miss:**
    - AAA rupture
    - Bowel rupture, perforation, ischemia
    - Ascending cholangitis
    - Acute appendicitis
    - Retroperitoneal hematoma

Key History:

Epigastrium:
Heart (MI, pericarditis, dissection)
AAA
Esophagus (GERD)
Stomach and duodenum (PUD, cancer)
Pancreas (pancreatitis, cancer)
Lung (PNA, PE)

Right upper quadrant:
Liver (hepatitis, perihepatits
Gallbladder (cholecystitis,
cholangitis, choledocho-
lithiasis)
Hepatic flexure (obstruction, cancer)
Lung (PNA, PE)

Left upper quadrant:
Spleen (rupture, infarct, abscess)
Splenic flexure
(obstruction, cancer)

Right lower quadrant:
Appendix (appendicitis, abscess)
Ovary (torsion, ruptured cyst, carcinoma)

Nephrolithiasis (flank to lower Quadrant to groin)

Left lower quadrant:
Left colon (diverticulitis,
Ischemic colitis, obstruction)
Ovary (torsion, ruptured cyst, carcinoma)

Hypogastrium:
Bladder (cystitis, obstruction)
Ovary (torsion, ruptured cyst, carcinoma)
Fallopian tubes (ectopic pregnancy, salpingitis, endometriosis)

- **Goal is to establish whether this is an acute abdomen or not**
- If vital signs are stable, it is most likely not urgent, and the patient does not need to be seen immediately
- How severe is the pain?
- Is this a new problem?
- What are the patient's vitals?
- What was the patient admitted for?
- Location of pain?
- Quality of pain?
    - Somatic pain is pinpoint
    - Visceral pain is vague
    - Neuropathic pain is burning or pins and needles
- Duration of pain?
- Radiation of pain?
- Pain that changes with respiration?
- N/V?
- Last bowel movement?
- Hematemesis?
- Melena?
- Hematochezia?
- LMP if female
- If Hx of A-fib and pain out of proportion to exam, think mesenteric ischemia
- Quickly review the chart and assess toxicity of the patient

Focused Examination:

- General: is the patient distressed or ill appearing?
- Vitals: repeat now, especially BP
- HEENT: check for icterus
- Chest:
    - Check for any skin lesions
    - Listen for murmur, rubs, or gallops

- Respiratory:
    - Assess JVP
    - Listen for crackles, absent breath sounds on one side, friction rub
- Abdomen:
    - Auscultate bowel sounds
        - High pitched with small bowel obstruction
        - Absent with ileus
    - Percussion:
        - Tympany
        - Shifting dullness
    - Palpation:
        - Guarding, rebound tenderness
        - Murphy's sign
        - Psoas sign and obturator signs
        - CVA tenderness
        - Pulsatile mass (AAA)
- Rectal:
    - Assess for hemorrhoids and anal fissures
    - Guiac for occult blood
- Pelvic:
    - If indicated by history

Labs/Diagnostics:

- CBC
- CMP
    - Electrolytes, LFTs, BUN/Cr
- Amylase
- Lipase
- Lactate
- Beta-HCG if female
- UA
- Possible CXR
- Possible EKG
- Abdominal CT, ultrasound, or both may be required

Management:

- Initial goal is to determine if the patient has an acute abdomen, and needs surgical evaluation and treatment:
    - An acute abdomen has rebound tenderness or guarding (especially involuntary)
    - Ruptured viscus, abscess, or hemorrhage are acute
- Other conditions can be managed using a more detailed approach after the acute abdomen has been ruled out
- Keep patient NPO
- Ensure IV access is present

Headache

Differential:

- Primary headache:
  - Tension
  - Migraine
  - Cluster
  - Analgesic rebound
- Secondary headache (has red flag signs/symptoms- see below):
  - Bleed
  - Infection
  - Tumor
  - Vasculitis (temporal arteritis)
  - Increased ICP
  - Severe hypertension
  - CVA
  - Infectious (meningitis, sinusitis)
- **Things you do not want to miss:**
  - Meningitis
  - Subarachnoid hemorrhage
  - Subdural hematoma
  - Epidural hematoma
  - Mass lesion with herniation

Key History:

- **If the headache is severe and acute or associated with N/V, changes in vision, other focal CNS findings, fever, or decreased consciousness, the patient should be seen ASAP**
- Check BP, pulse, respirations, O2 sats, and temperature
- How severe is the headache?
- Has there been a change in consciousness?
- Are there any new focal neurological deficits?
- Has the patient had similar headaches in the past? If so, what precipitates or relieves them?
- Quickly look at the patient and review the chart
- **Red flags:**
  - Fever
  - Focal neurological deficits
  - Age >40 and new headache
  - Positional headache
  - Seizure

Focused Examination:

- General: does the patient appear ill or distressed?
- HEENT:
  - Look for signs of trauma
  - Pupil size/symmetry response to light
  - Papilledema
  - Nuchal rigidity
  - Temporal artery tenderness
  - Sinus tenderness
- Neurological:
  - Thorough exam is mandatory

o   Mental status exam

Labs/Diagnostics:

- If temporal arteritis suspected, consider CBC and ESR
- **Head CT** should be considered for:
    o   A chronic headache pattern that has changed or a new severe headache occurs
    o   A new headache in a patient older than 40
    o   Focal findings on neurological exam
- If meningitis suspected, an LP should be performed
    o   Do not need to do a CT before LP if the patient is non-elderly (<60), immunocompetent, no focal neurological abnormalities, seizures, or diminished level of consciousness

Management:

- **Initial goal is to exclude the serious life-threatening conditions mentioned previously**
- Management for non life-threatening conditions focuses on symptomatic relief
- For **suspected bacterial meningitis**, start antibiotics (ceftriaxone + vancomycin), dexamethasone before antibiotics
- For **suspected subdural/epidural hematoma or subarachnoid hemorrhage**, obtain CT scan, if positive, neurosurgery consult
- **Tension headaches and mild migraines** can be treated with acetaminophen or ibuprofen; consider sumatriptan for moderate to severe migraines
- **Severe migraines** may require an opiate; sumatriptan and ergotamine are usually effective in the prodromal stage

Hypotension

Differential:

- Cardiogenic (rate or pump problem)
- Hypovolemic
- Septic shock
- Anaphylaxis
- **Things you do not want to miss:**
    o   Shock is inadequate tissue and organ perfusion. This is best addressed by looking at end organs:
        ▪ Brain (mental status)
        ▪ Heart (chest pain)
        ▪ Kidneys (urine output)
        ▪ Skin (cool, clammy)
    o   Shock is a clinical diagnosis with SBP <90 with evidence of inadequate tissue perfusion

Key History:

- **Hypotension requires that you see the patient ASAP**
- What are the vital signs?

- Is the patient conscious, confused, or disoriented?
- What has the BP been?
- What was the reason for admission?
- Any potential of blood loss?
- IV access?
- Check BP in both arms, pulse, respirations, O2 sats, temperature
- Quickly review patient chart

Focused Examination:

- General: how distressed or sick does the patient look?
- Vitals: repeat now and often
    - Elevated temperature and hypotension suggest sepsis
- Cardiovascular:
    - Heart rate, JVP, skin temperature, color, warmth, capillary refill
- Lungs:
    - Listen for crackles, breath sounds on both sides
- GI:
    - Any evidence of blood loss?
- Neurologic:
    - Mentation, symmetric movements

Labs/Diagnostics:

- Consider troponins, EKG, ABG, CBC, electrolytes, CXR

Management:

- Examine EKG and take the pulse yourself
    - Look for atrial fibrillation, SVT, ventricular tachycardia
    - These may cause hypotension because of decreased diastolic filling
- A compensatory sinus tachycardia is expected in hypotension
- Bradycardia may occur in autonomic dysfunction or heart block
- Check BP in both arms
- **Fluids** to normalize intravascular volume, especially in shock
    - Use normal saline or lactated Ringers
    - **Exception is cardiogenic shock**, which may require preload and afterload reduction, inotropic and/or vasopressor support, and transfer to an ICU
- Hypovolemic, anaphylactic, and septic shock require fluids
    - Use boluses of 500 mL to 1 L, and repeat if no response
- **Anaphylactic shock requires epinephrine**, 0.3 mg IV immediately and repeated every 10-15 minutes as required
    - Hydrocortisone and diphenhydramine should also be administered
    - Glucocorticoids do nothing for emergent symptoms, but are given to prevent prolonged or recurrent anaphylactic reactions
- **Septic shock requires fluids and antibiotics**
    - Continuing hypotension requires ICU admission for vasopressors
- **Cardiogenic shock** can be the result of an acute MI or worsening CHF
    - Other causes of hypotension and elevated JVP should be ruled out (acute cardiac tamponade, PE, and tension pneumothorax)

Hypertension

Differential:

- **Hypertensive emergency and urgency are what you need to worry about acutely in the hospital with BP**
- Hypertensive **Emergency**:
    o Severe elevations of blood pressure in the presence of acute end-organ damage (>180/>120)
    o End organ damage signs:
        - Encephalopathy
        - Intracranial hemorrhage
        - Unstable angina or MI (elevated troponins)
        - Acute LV failure with pulmonary edema
        - Aortic dissection
        - Eclampsia
        - Renal insufficiency (new or worsened)
- Hypertensive **Urgency**:
    o Severe elevations of blood pressure without the presence of acute end-organ damage (diastolic BP >120-130)
    o Optic disc edema
    o Severe perioperative hypertension
- **Things you do not want to miss:**
    o Hypertensive emergencies with acute end organ system damage

Key History:

- What are the vitals?
- What has the patients BP been?
- What is the reason for admission?
- What BP meds has the patient been taking?
- Are they confused, have decreased urine output, or have chest pain?
- **The rate of rise of the BP is more important than the BP itself**
- Quickly review chart

Focused Examination:

- General: is the patient distressed or ill appearing?
- Vitals: repeat BP in **both arms**
- HEENT:
    o Check fundi for papilledema, retinal hemorrhages, or other hypertensive changes
- Cardiovascular:
    o HR, JVP, capillary refill
- Respiratory:
    o Listen for crackles, breath sounds on both sides
- Neurologic:
    o Mentation, confusion, delirium, focal neurologic deficits

Labs/Diagnostics:

- Consider troponins, EKG, ABG, CBC, electrolytes, UA, and CXR

Management:

- **Treat the patient, NOT the BP**
    - Acute lowering of BP in asymptomatic patients with long-standing hypertension can be dangerous
- Permissive hypertension is usually advised by neurologists for patients with an acute ischemic stroke, unless the BP is severely elevated (>220/120) or conditions such as acute coronary syndrome, decompensated CHF, aortic dissection, encephalopathy, acute renal failure, and eclampsia coexist
- **Hypertensive emergencies require an ICU setting**
    - The goal is to reduce MAP by no more than 25% in the first 2 hours
    - IV hydralazine, nitroprusside, labetalol, esmolol, enalaprilate, and fenoldopm are often used
    - If MR or pulmonary edema, consider IV nitroglycerin
    - If aortic dissection, nitroprusside and labetalol
- **Hypertensive urgencies can usually be managed with oral medications**
    - Goal of reducing BP over 24-48 hours
    - Examples include captopril 25-50 mg PO, clonidine 0.1-0.2 mg PO, or labetalol 200-400mg PO, these can be repeated or titrated every 2-4 hours
    - Close follow up is essential

Conditions	Preferred Antihypertensive Agents
Acute pulmonary edema/systolic dysfunction	Nicardipine, fenoldopam, or nitroprusside in combination with nitroglycerin and a loop diuretic
Acute pulmonary edema/diastolic dysfunction	Esmolol, metoprolol, labetalol, or verapamil in combination with low-dose nitroglycerin and a loop diuretic
Acute myocardial ischemia	Labetalol or esmolol in combination with nitroglycerin
Hypertensive encephalopathy	Nicardipine, labetalol, or fenoldopam
Acute aortic dissection	Lebatalol or combination of niardipine and esmolol or combination of nitroprusside and either esmolol or IV metoprolol
Pre-eclampsia, eclampsia	Labetalol or nicardipine
Acute renal failure/microangiopathic anemia	Nicardipine or fenoldopam
Sympathetic crisis/cocaine overdose	Verapamil, diltiazem, or nicardipine in combination with a benzodiazepine
Acute ischemic stroke/intracerebral bleed	Nicardipine, labetalol, or fenoldopam

Common Arrhythmias

Differential:

- Rapid rates, regular rhythm:
    - Sinus tachycardia
    - SVT

- Ventricular tachycardia
    - Atrial flutter
- Rapid rates, irregular rhythm:
    - Atrial fibrillation with rapid ventricular rate
    - Multifocal atrial tachycardia
- Slow rates:
    - Drugs (beta blockers, CCB, digoxin)
    - Sick sinus syndrome
    - MI (especially inferior)
    - AV block
- **Things you do not want to miss:**
    - Ventricular tachycardia
    - Unstable SVT
    - Hypotension
    - Angina or MI

Key History:

- **Patients with chest pain, SOB, altered mental status, or hypotension need to be seen ASAP**
- What are the vitals?
- Any chest pain or SOB?
- What is the patient's mental status?
- Quickly look at patient and review chart while waiting for EKG

Focused Examination:

- General: does the patient look sick or distressed?
- Vitals: repeat now
- Cardiovascular:
    - HR, JVP
    - Skin temperature and color
    - Capillary refill
- Respiratory:
    - Listen for crackles and breath sounds on both sides
- Neurologic:
    - Evaluate for confusion or change in level of consciousness

Labs/Diagnostics:

- EKG
- Consider troponins, ABG, CBC, electrolytes, and CXR

Management:

- **Always complete ABCs first and ensure O2 and IV access**
- Place on monitor or telemetry; consider transfer to higher level of care if needed
- **Cardioversion** may be required if the patient is hypotensive and has atrial fibrillation with RVR, SVT, or ventricular tachycardia

- If patient is **unstable** with serious signs or symptoms (chest pain, SOB, decreased consciousness, hypotension and shock, CHF, acute MI), a ventricular rate of > 150, or both, prepare for immediate cardioversion
- Patient may require sedation before cardioversion
- **A-fib with RVR** that is hemodynamically **stable** can be controlled with diltiazem, metoprolol, esmolol, or digoxin
    - Amiodarone can be considered, and is the best choice if heart failure and/or an accessory pathway is present
    - Diltiazem 0.25 mg/kg IVP over 2 minutes; if no response, 0.35 mg/kg IVP over 2 minutes and follow with an IV infusion at 5-15 mg/h
    - Metoprolol 2.5-5mg IVP over 2 minutes every 5 minutes to a total of 15 mg followed by oral dosing; **best choice if ischemia is suspected or present**
    - Esmolol 0.5 mg/kg over 1 minute loading dose, followed by 50 mcg/kg/min, max 300 mcg/kg/min
    - Digoxin 0.25-0.5 mg IVP, then 0.125-0.25 mg IVP every 4-6 hours to a total dose of 0.75-1.35 mg; slower effect, may be used in CHF
    - Amiodarone 150mg IV over 10 minutes, followed by infusion of 1mg/min for 6 hours, then 0.5 mg/min for 18 hours
- **SVT** that is hemodynamically **stable** can sometimes be broke with Valsalva maneuver, carotid sinus massage (listen for bruits first, do only one side at a time)
    - If still in SVT, try adenosine 6 mg rapid IV push followed by 12 mg rapid IV push if necessary (remember to flush with at least 20 mL NS after each IV push)
- For V-tach that is pulseless or without BP, manage as V-fib using ACLS protocol

Fever

Differential:

- Infections:
    - Lung
    - Urine
    - IV sites
    - Blood/cardiac
    - CNS
    - Abdomen
    - Pelvis
- Drug induced fever:
    - Antibiotics and many other drugs
- Postoperative atelectasis
- Neoplasms
- Rheumatologic diseases
- DVT/PE
- Fever of unknown origin
- **Things you do not want to miss:**
    - Meningitis
    - Septic shock, particularly in neutropenic patients
    - Endocarditis

Key History:

- **Patients with symptoms concerning for meningitis, and immunocompromised patients need to be seen ASAP**
- What are the patient's vitals?
- What was the reason for admission?
- Is this a new finding?
- Any associated symptoms?
    - Cough
    - Headache
    - Change in mental status
    - N/V
- Any antipyretics or current antibiotics?
- Any recent surgeries or procedures?

Focused Examination:

- General: Does the patient appear ill? Check all catheter sites (IV, central line, Foley, G-tube, etc.)
- Vitals: repeat now, tachycardia is an expected finding with fever
- Cardiovascular:
    - HR, JVP
    - Skin temperature and color
    - Any new murmurs?
    - Capillary refill
- Respiratory:
    - Listen for crackles and breath sounds on both sides
- Abdomen:
    - Assess for localized tenderness and bowel sounds
- Extremities:
    - Check calves for signs of DVT and joints for effusions
- Neurologic:
    - Mentation
    - Photophobia
    - Neck stiffness
    - Brudzinski or Kernigs sign

Labs/Diagnostics:

- Consider CBC, blood cultures (two sets at different sites, if central line present get one from there and get one at a peripheral site as well), CMP, UA and culture, sputum culture and Gram's stain, CXR
- LP if meningitis suspected
- Fluid collections (ie pleural effusions, ascites) may need tapped
- Consider C. diff toxin stool testing

Management:

- Make sure patient is hemodynamically stable
- Review medications and obtain cultures

- Give antipyretics (acetaminophen 650 mg PO or ibuprofen 500 mg PO Q6-8h prn)
- Ensure IV access and consider maintenance fluids for insensible losses
- Consider antibiotics carefully
    o If the patient is stable, immunocompetent, not toxic appearing, with no clear source of infection, it may be prudent to withhold antibiotics and await culture results
    o Fever and hypotension requires broad spectrum antibiotics and IV fluids or pressors to manage the hypotension
- Patient with fever and meningitis symptoms require antibiotics immediately, do not wait for the LP to be done
- Consider changing or removing foley catheters and any indwelling IV sites
- **Febrile neutropenia:**
    o Fever of >38.3C with ANC $\leq$ 500
    o **Cefepime** 1 g IV Q8h to begin
        ▪ If PCN allergy, give ciprofloxacin 400 mg IV Q 12h or aztreonam 2 g IV Q8h
    o Vancomycin 1 g IV Q12h if any of the following are present: severe mucositis, evidence of catheter related infection, known colonization with resistant staph or strep, sudden temperature spike > 40C, hypotension, or sepsis
    o Consider metronidazole 500 mg IV Q8h if suspected oropharyngeal or intra-abdominal source
    o Consider gentamicin 5 mg/kg IV Q 24h X 72 h if clinically unstable

Shortness of Breath

Differential:

- Pulmonary:
    o Asthma
    o COPD
    o PE
    o Pneumonia
    o Pleural effusion
- Cardiovascular:
    o CHF
    o MI/ischemia
    o Cardiac tamponade
    o Arrhythmias
- Others;
    o Pneumothorax
    o Obstruction (mucous plug)
    o Anxiety
- **Things you do not want to miss:**
    o Inadequate tissue oxygenation (hypoxia)
    o Tension pneumothorax
    o Airway obstruction
    o PE

Key History:

- **Patients with SOB need to be seen ASAP**
- What are the patient's vitals?
- When was the onset of SOB and what was the reason for admission?
- Does the patient have a history of asthma or COPD?
- Is the patient getting oxygen?
- Quickly look at the patient and review the chart
- Get an EKG and CXR if the patient looks sick

Focused Examination:

- General: does the patient appear ill or distressed?
- Vitals: repeat now, check for pulsus paradoxus
- Cardiovascular:
    - HR, JVP
    - Skin temperature and color
    - Capillary refill
- Respiratory:
    - Listen for crackles and breath sounds on both sides
    - Evidence of consolidation or effusion
- Neurologic:
    - Mentation

Labs/Diagnostics:

- Consider ABG, EKG, troponins, D-dimer, CTA, and CXR
- If you have any doubt at all, get an ABG

Management:

- Supplemental O2 to keep SaO2 > 92%
    - Be cautious if they have COPD and retain CO2, then do SaO2 88-92%
- Asthma or COPD:
    - Albuterol and ipratropium (**Duoneb**) by nebulizer, Q2-4h until stable
    - Consider IV methylprednisolone 60 mg IV Q6h, and antibiotics if needed
- For CHF:
    - If patient is volume overloaded, raise head of bed and give Lasix 20-40 mg IV and albuterol nebulizer
    - Consider nitroglycerin or morphine
    - Assess for adequate diuresis
- For suspected cardiac tamponade, order a stat cardiac echo or do bedside ultrasound and cardiology consult
- For PE:
    - Patient is tachycardic and tachypneic and has a sudden onset of SOB
    - EKG shows sinus tachycardia most commonly, can show S1Q3T3
    - If suspicion high, consider starting heparin or lovenox
    - Obtain CT angiogram or a V/Q scan

- Acute respiratory failure:
    - Defined by ABG of PO2 <60 or PCO2 >50 with a pH of < 7.3 on room air
    - Ensure patient has not received narcotics recently, if so consider naloxone 0.2 mg IV
    - If respiratory failure with pH < 7.2, intubation is usually required

GI Bleeding

Differential:

- Upper GI bleed:
    - Esophageal varices
    - Mallory Weiss tear
    - Peptic ulcer
    - Esophagitis
    - Neoplasm
    - Aortoenteric fistula (history of AAA repair)
- Lower GI bleed:
    - Diverticulosis
    - Angiodysplasia
    - Neoplasm
    - Inflammatory bowel disease
    - Infectious colitis
    - Anorectal disease (hemorrhoids, fissures)
- **Things you do not want to miss:**
    - GI bleeding leading to hypovolemic shock

Key History:

- **If the patient is tachycardic or hypotensive, see the patient ASAP**
- What are the patient's vitals?
- When was the onset of bleeding and what is the reason for admission?
- Is the bleeding upper (coffee ground emesis, melena) or lower (hematochezia)?
- How much blood has been lost?
- Quickly look at the patient and review the chart

Focused Examination:

- General: how distressed or sick does the patient look?
- Vitals: repeat now
- HEENT:
    - Check for conjunctival pallor or scleral icterus
- Cardiovascular:
    - HR, JVP
    - Skin temperature and color
    - Capillary refill
- Abdomen:
    - Check for tenderness and bowel sounds
    - Look for ascites
- Rectal:

- Must be performed
- Guiac stool
- Neurologic:
  - Evaluate level of consciousness and ability to protect airway

Labs/Diagnostics:

- Consider CBC, coags, and CMP
- The initial CBC may be deceptive in acute GI bleeding

Management:

- Insert two large bore IV (16-18G)
- Type and cross PRBCs
- Stop anticoagulation if on any, and consider reversal with FFP or vitamin K
- Consider whether the patient needs premedication with acetaminophen/diphenhydramine based on prior transfusions
- Bolster the intravascular volume by giving IV fluids (NS), especially while waiting for blood products
- NPO
- **For Upper GI bleeding:**
  - Insert NG tube with lavage to assess if active bleeding is present
  - PPI drip or IV PPI therapy
  - GI consult for endoscopy
- **For active variceal bleeding in patients with cirrhosis:**
  - **IV octreotide** 50 mcg bolus, then 50 mcg/h
    - Can be life saving
  - IV ceftriaxone 1g/day
  - Correct coagulation deficits
  - Replace PRBCs as needed
  - Call GI consult for endoscopy
- **For lower GI bleeding:**
  - Correct fluid status
  - If stable, obtain GI consult for colonoscopy
  - If unstable, an urgent tagged RBC scan should be scheduled
  - Consider arteriography
- Surgery consult/indications:
  - Aortoenteric fistula
  - Uncontrollable or recurrent bleeding
  - Bleeding episode requiring transfusion of more than 6 units PRBCs
  - Visible naked vessel seen in peptic ulcer by endoscopy

Common Diseases in Internal Medicine

Urinary Tract Infections

Definitions:

Complicated UTI- UTI's that have any of the following: male sex, diabetes, renal failure, pregnancy, history of pyelonephritis in the last year, urinary tract obstruction, indwelling catheter, stents, nephrostomy tube, antibiotic resistant organism, recent antibiotic use, recent hospitalization, and an immunocompromised patient. These may predispose to treatment failure and management changes due to resistant microorganisms.

History:

The history in urinary tract infections is used to determine many things. Whether this is a lower or upper UTI, an uncomplicated or complicated UTI, recurrent or first time, a known and preventable cause, catheter associated, STDs, and any other comorbidity that may be contributing to the infection. The answers to these questions will help guide treatment strategies acutely, and possibly chronically.

CC:

HPI:

- Character, Onset, Location, Intensity, Description, Duration, Exacerbating factors, Relieving factors, Radiation, associated Signs/symptoms
    - *From now on,* **COLIDDERRS**, *or use any mnemonic you like*
    - *Cystitis- urgency, frequency, dysuria*
    - *Pyelonephritis- urgency, frequency, dysuria, n/v, CVA tenderness, fever*
    - *Perinephric abscess- pyelonephritis that does not get better*
- Fever/chills?
    - *Signs of sepsis and fever can indicate an upper UTI*
- Nausea/vomiting?
    - *May not be able to swallow oral antibiotics, sign of upper UTI*
- Recurrent?
    - *May be able to look up old culture susceptibilities, may change treatment plan, may need to use preventative strategies for future*
- Flank pain?
    - *May show it is a pyelonephritis or kidney stone*
- Suprapubic tenderness?
    - *Sign of a cystitis*
- Dysuria?
    - *Sign of any type of UTI*
- Hematuria?
    - *Sign of any type of UTI*
- Urinary urgency?
    - *Sign of any type of UTI or STD*
- Urinary frequency?

- - *Sign of any type of UTI*
- Vaginal discharge?
  - *Sign of any type of UTI or STD*
- Catheter?
  - *Makes it a complicated UTI*
- Sexual activity?
  - Does the sexual partner have symptoms?
  - *STD screening and honeymoon cystitis*
- Current/prior STD's?
- Last menses?
  - *Can help explain blood in urine if present*

ROS:

PMH:

- Prior UTI's?
  - *Can help with initial antibiotic to use, previous cultures, resistant organisms*
- Hx of STD's?
  - *Can help with initial antibiotic to use, previous cultures, resistant organisms*
- Hx of Diabetes?
  - *Makes it complicated and may be prone to pseudomonas and candida*
- Hx of Neurological diseases → incontinence
  - *Full bladder and incomplete emptying can make susceptible to UTIs*
- Urogenital anatomic abnormalities?
  - *Makes it complicated*

Surgical H:

- Urogenital surgeries?
  - *Makes it complicated and more prone*

Social H:

- Alcohol, smoking, recreational drugs, job, living situation
- **Sexual history**

Family H:

Allergies:

Medications:

Canagliflozin (invokana) and dapagliflozin (farxiga) are SGLT2 inhibitors that make patients prone to UTIs.

Physical Examination:

The physical examination should focus on vital signs, mental status, respiratory, cardiac, abdominal, genital, and signs of dehydration. It is important to determine whether this is a lower or upper UTI, as well as if signs of severe sepsis or septic shock are present, indicating urosepsis.

- Vitals signs
    - Fever can indicate upper UTI
    - Hypotension can indicate severe sepsis or septic shock
    - Tachycardia and tachypnea
    - Hypertension could be a sign of chronic kidney damage
- Mental status
    - Many urosepsis patients will have signs of altered mental status, and could be the main symptom in the presentation if the person is unable to voice typical UTI symptoms
- Oral mucosa for moist or dehydration
- Respiratory exam
- Cardiac exam
- Abdominal exam
    - Suprapubic pain (lower or upper UTI)
    - CVA tenderness (upper UTI)
- Genital exam
    - Catheter
    - Genital lesions
    - Bimanual exam if indicated
        - Anterior vaginal pain with palpation if cystitis/urethritis
- Volume status

Differential Diagnosis:

- Cystitis
    - *Suprapubic pain, dysuria, possible hematuria, less likely to have fever, no flank pain*
- Pyelonephritis
    - *CVA tenderness with fever and other common UTI symptoms (dysuria, frequency, hematuria, etc.)*
- STD's
    - *Have dysuria, genital pus/discharge, typical lesions of STD's, recent sexual activity*
- Epididymitis
    - *Gradual onset (days) of scrotal pain and swelling, unilateral, dysuria, frequency, fever and chills in some, urethral discharge preceding pain in some cases*
- Prostatitis
    - *Fever, chills, arthralgias, perineal/prostatic pain, dysuria, obstructive urinary tract symptoms, low back/abdominal pain*
- Pelvic inflammatory disease
    - *Young female with recent sexual intercourse, fever, nausea, vomiting, lower abdominal pain that is dull, achy, or crampy and constant bilaterally, exacerbated by movement, vaginal discharge*
- Ectopic pregnancy

- o *Lower abdominal pain, amenorrhea, vaginal bleeding, fever, and possibly abdominal rigidity, involuntary guarding, and evidence of hypovolemic shock*
- Perinephric abscess
    - o *Fever 1-2 weeks after UTI with unilateral flank pain, nonspecific symptoms, diagnosed with US or CT*
- Nephrolithiasis
    - o *Flank pain radiating to the inguinal area, dysuria, no fever*

Labs:

- CBC with differential
    - o Look for leukocytosis, anemia
- BMP
    - o Look for electrolyte abnormalities, hyperglycemia
- Beta-HCG if female
- Blood cultures if sepsis, **before antibiotics**
- UA with urine cultures
    - o Nitrites, leukocyte esterase
    - o WBC's → most important
    - o Leukocyte casts → present in pyelonephritis
    - o Wet mount if considering chlamydia or gonorrhea
    - o If squamous epithelial cells are present, it is **contaminated**, get another
    - o Can have hematuria
- **Previous urine cultures if available**
    - o Helps with choice of initial empiric antibiotic treatment

Imaging:

- If suspected cystitis → none
- If suspected pyelonephritis → US
- Consider CT abdomen/pelvis if complicated/septic shock, or if not improving in 48-72 hours

Treatment:

Inpatient:

- Admit patient if have sepsis, complicated UTI, altered mental status, etc.
- **If prior urine cultures available, tailor initial therapy based off those susceptibilities**
- Empiric treatment:
    - o Ceftriaxone IV 1g Q24h
    - o Ciprofloxacin 500mg ER PO Q24h X3 days if uncomplicated, 1000mg ER PO Q24h X7 days if complicated
    - o Bactrim 1 DS (160/800mg) PO X3-14 days
- **Tailor therapies as soon as culture susceptibilities come back**, usually treat for total of 7 days if was hospitalized with cystitis, or 14 days if pyelonephritis
- **Risk factors for multi-drug resistant organisms:**
    - o Current or recent hospitalization
    - o Immunocompromised

- Presence of underlying structural abnormalities
- Previous UTI
- Kidney transplantation
- Recent antimicrobial therapy

Outpatient:

- For acute uncomplicated cystitis/pyelonephritis
- Bactrim 1 DS PO X 5 days
- Nitrofurantoin 1000mg PO BID X 5days
- Fosfomycin 3g single dose (not as affective and more expensive)
- For pyelonephritis → ciprofloxacin 500mg PO BID X 7 days, or levofloxacin 750mg PO X 5-7 days
- Phenazopyridine 100-200mg PO TID x 2 days for urinary analgesia
- Prophylaxis:
    - If at least 3 UTI in one year, or 2 in a 6 month period
    - **Women with a history of acute cystitis can recognize the symptoms of UTI recurrence and provide appropriate self-treatment**
    - Bactrim/nitrofurantoin after intercourse or with recognition of symptoms
    - Low dose Bactrim for 6 months

Asymptomatic bacteriuria should NOT be treated UNLESS they are pregnant or before urologic procedures

Etiology:

Uncomplicated UTI:

- **E. coli** (75-90%)
- Staphylococcus saprophyticus
- Klebsiella
- Proteus
    - Increased urine pH
- Enterococcus
- Citrobacter

Complicated UTI:

- **E. coli** still most common cause
- Pseudomonas
- Klebsiella
- Proteus
- Citrobacter
- Acinetobacter
- Morganella
- Candida

Risk Factors:

- Female
- Recent sexual intercourse
    - Seprmicide and diaphragm use
    - Anal intercourse
- Congenital urinary tract abnormalities
- BPH
- Diabetes
- Incontinence
- Pregnancy
- Catheter
- Postmenopausal
- Vaginal infection
- Obesity
- Uncircumcised

Pathogenesis:

- Ascending bacteria from urethra migrate to the bladder
- Interplay of environment, hygiene, bacteria, and host immunodeficiency
- Vesicoureteral reflux for pyelonephritis

Complications:

- Pyelonephritis
- Emphysematous pyelonephritis **(especially in diabetics)**
- Xanthogranulomatous pyelonephritis
- Intraparenchymal abscess
- Chronic pyelonephritis with scarring
- Sepsis to septic shock

Admission Orders:

- Admit to floor
- Diagnosis cystitis/pyelonephritis/complicated/uncomplicated
- Condition stable/guarded
- Vital signs routine
- Allergies
- Activity ad lib
- Nursing routine- Call for T >38.5, Systolic BP <100, HR >110
- Diet clear liquids until tolerating PO, then advance diet
- Fluid resuscitation
- Meds:
    - Ceftriaxone IV 1g Q24h
    - Zofran 4mg IV Q4-6h prn
- Labs/diagnostics:
    - UA with culture
    - CBC
    - BMP

- o Blood cultures if septic
- o Beta-HCG if female
- o Gram stain and culture if indicated
- o If suspected pyelonephritis → US
- o CT early if sepsis, complicated UTI, or UTI not improving after 48-72 hours

Discharge Information:

- Able to tolerate PO food and medications
- Treat for 10-14 days and perform f/u urine culture outpatient

Additional Notes:

- <u>Treatment in pregnancy</u>- nitrofurantoin, ampicillin, amoxicillin, and cephalosporins are safe. Avoid sulfonamides and fluoroquinolones

Pneumonia

Definitions:

Community acquired pneumonia- pneumonia acquired before hospitalization, or within 72 hours of being hospitalized.

Hospital acquired pneumonia- pneumonia acquired after 72 hours of being hospitalized.

History:

It is important to know about comorbidities and prior medical conditions when considering pneumonia. CHF and COPD exacerbation may present like pneumonia. Aspiration pneumonia may occur in certain populations such as alcoholics, patients prone to seizures, and patients with neurological conditions. Chest pain can also be a symptom of pneumonia, making acute coronary syndrome a possibility that needs to be ruled out. Immunocompromised states, such as HIV, also has to be considered as treatment will change. Cystic fibrosis patients are very susceptible. There are regional patterns to certain infections, such as coccidiomycosis, histoplasmosis, blastomycosis, and aspergillus.

CC:

HPI:

- COLIDDERRS
  - *Typical pneumonias have acute onset of fever, shaking chills, thick productive cough, pleuritic chest pain, dyspnea*
  - *Atypical pneumonias have insidious onset with headache, sore throat, fatigue, myalgias, nonproductive cough, fevers without chills (chills uncommon)*
  - *In the end it **does not matter if it is typical or atypical, it DOES matter if it is CAP, HCAP, HAP, or VAP***
- Fever/chills?
  - *Part of CURB-65 and common symptom of pneumonia*
- Cough?
  - Productive? Hemoptysis?
  - *Common symptom, plus quality helps with possible PE, vs infectious*
- SOB?
- Chest pain?
  - Pleuritic?
  - *Pleuritic more likely pneumonia than acute coronary syndrome*
- Sinus pain?
  - *Helps rule out sinusitis*
- Recent illness?
  - *Recent viral illness predisposes to pneumonias, especially with S. aureus*
- Nausea/vomiting?
  - *Common symptom of pneumonia and may not be able to take oral antibiotics*
- Edema?
  - *Can help if CHF is a possibility*

- Recent trauma?
  - *Could have pneumothorax or hemothorax*
- Change in mental status?
  - *Part of CURB-65*
- Smoker?
  - *More susceptible to pneumonia*
- Recent antibiotic use?
  - Important in terms of what antibiotics you may use, especially in the outpatient setting
- Diarrhea?
  - Legionella produces diarrhea with pneumonia and relative bradycardia

ROS:

PMH:

- Hx of CHF?
  - *CHF produces SOB and can help you determine between pneumonia and CHF exacerbation*
- Hx of COPD?
  - *Might lean you towards a COPD exacerbation, but they are more prone to pneumonias, and may be infected with a COPD exacerbation and pneumonia*
- Hx of HIV/AIDS?
  - *Pneumocystitis jiroveci pneumonia should be on the differential*
- Hx of Cystic fibrosis?
  - *More likely to have pseudomonas or S. aureus pneumonias*
- Hx of Neurological disease?
  - *More prone to aspiration pneumonia from anaerobes*
- Prior radiation?
  - *Can have radiation pneumonitis if recent, but also likely to have cancer*
- Hx of Sarcoidosis?
  - *Prone to cough, as well as pneumonias*

Surgical H:

Social H:

- Alcohol, smoking, recreational drugs, job, living situation, sexual
- **Where is the patient from regionally**
  - *Histoplasmosis in the Mississippi and Ohio River Valleys*
  - *Blastomycosis in states east of the Mississippi river and in Central America*
  - *Coccidiomycosis in Southwestern states and California*
  - *Paracoccidiomycosis in Latin America*

Family H:

Allergies:

Medications:

Antibiotics within the last 3 months can change treatment.

Physical Examination:

Obviously the respiratory exam is important in pneumonia. Vital signs are important in not only diagnosing sepsis, but also to consider whether the patient can be treated outpatient, or needs to be admitted to the floor or to the ICU. Mental status is important as well. The cardiac exam is important as it can help differentiate pneumonia and CHF.

- Vital signs
    - Tachypnea and BP part of CURB-65 (see below)
- Lymphadenopathy
- Oral mucosa moist or dry
- Cardiac
    - S3 can indicate CHF
    - New murmur may indicate an MI
    - JVD (RHF)
- Respiratory
    - RR, accessory muscle use, tactile fremitus, dullness to percussion (consolidation), crackles
- Abdominal
    - Pain, hepatomegaly (can indicate RHF)
- Mental status exam

Differential Diagnosis:

- Non-infectious:
    - CHF
        - *Cardiac history, no fever, edema*
    - PE
        - *Tachycardia, less or no edema, hemoptysis*
    - Radiation pneumonitis
        - *History of lung cancer/radiation*
    - COPD exacerbation
        - *History of lung disease/COPD/smoker*
    - Cancer
    - Sarcoidosis
        - *African American female with bilateral hilar lymphadenopathy, possibly erythema nodosum present*
    - Aspiration
        - *Alcoholic, seizure, neurological disease with trouble eating*
- Infectious:
    - Acute bronchitis
        - *No CXR findings, hemoptysis*
    - URI
        - *More nasal/sinus symptoms*
    - Abscess
        - *See on CXR, sick for a long time*
    - Empyema

- *See on CXR, sick for a long time*
- Coccidiomycosis
  - *In Southwestern states and California*
- Histoplasmosis
  - *In the Mississippi and Ohio River Valleys*
- Blastomycosis
  - *In states east of the Mississippi river and in Central America*
- Aspergillus
- Bronchiectasis
  - *Chronic cough, recurrent or chronic pneumonia, foul smelling sputum, hemoptysis*

Labs:

- Sputum culture and gram stain if indicated (ICU admission, pleural effusion present, cavitary lesions on CXR)
  - For eventual specific antibiotic therapies
- **Blood cultures before antibiotics**
  - Need to see if bacteremia is present
- CBC with differential
  - Presence of leukocytosis
- BMP
  - Diarrhea with pneumonia and bradycardia who also has **hyponatremia, consider legionella**
  - Glucose, need to treat if hyperglycemic
- Troponins if considering ischemia as a source of SOB
- BNP
  - Possibly rule out CHF
- UA with culture if altered mental status
  - Possible UTI sepsis causing lung infiltrates
- Urinary Ag test for legionella/strep if indicated (smokers, elderly, immunocompromised, patients being considered for ICU)
- PCR for viruses, mycoplasma, and mycobacteria if indicated (same as for legionella/strep)
- CRP
- Procalcitonin
  - Increased with bacterial pneumonias as cells release procalcitonin in response to bacterial toxins, it is decreased or normal in viral pneumonias

Imaging:

- CXR
  - Typical pneumonia
    - Lobar consolidation
    - Multilobar consolidation is serious disease
  - Atypical pneumonia
    - Diffuse reticulonodular infiltrates
    - Absent or minimal consolidation
- CT chest if suspected postobstructive pneumonia from a tumor or foreign body or cavitary lesion, or not improving after 72 hours of antibiotics

- EKG
    - To rule out a cardiac cause of either chest pain or SOB that can be associated with a pneumonia

Prognostic Factors and Admission Criteria:

Pneumonia Severity Index:

- 20 criteria, separated into different classes
- Class 3 and above can be admitted
- **This is used by IM doctors**

CURB-65:

- 1 point for each
    - Confusion
    - Urea $\geq$ 20
    - RR $\geq$ 30
    - Systolic BP $\leq$ 90 or diastolic BP $\leq$ 60
    - Age $\geq$ 65
- A score of 2 → admit to floor
- $\geq$ 3 → admit to ICU
- 2= 9.2% mortality, $\geq$ 3= 33% mortality
- **This is used by ED doctors**

Treatment:

Core Measures:

- Cultures before antibiotics
- First dose of antibiotics in the ED
- Oxygen assessment (SpO2, ABG)
- Smoking cessation
- Vaccines

Empiric Inpatient Treatment:

- Non-ICU:
    - Respiratory fluoroquinolone or a beta lactam + a macrolide
        - Levofloxacin 750mg or moxifloxacin 400mg
        - Either **ceftriaxone**, ampicillin, cefotaxime, or ertapenem plus **azithromycin**, clarithromycin
    - Treat for 7 days, switch to oral meds once patient is clinically stable (afebrile, HR <100, RR <24, SaO2 >90% on room air, tolerating PO, normal mental status)
    - Once patient has met the above criteria and is on PO meds, no longer needs to be monitored in the hospital
- ICU:
    - Beta lactam + azithromycin or a respiratory fluoroquinolone
        - Either ceftriaxone, unasyn, zosyn, or cefotaxime plus either azithromycin, levofloxacin, or moxifloxacin

Empiric Outpatient Treatment:

- Previously healthy and no antibiotics within 3 months, <65, otherwise healthy:
    - Macrolide or doxycycline
        - Either azithromycin or clarithromycin, or
        - Doxycycline
- Comorbidities or antibiotics within 3 months, > 65:
    - Respiratory fluoroquinolone or beta lactam
        - Levofloxacin or moxifloxacin
        - High dose amoxicillin or augmentin (preferred)
        - Ceftriaxone, cefodoxime, cefuroxime + a macrolide

Special Considerations:

- Pseudomonas:
    - Antipseudomonal + ciprofloxacin or levofloxacin, or antipseudomonal + aminoglycoside + azithromycin, or antipseudmonal + aminoglycoside + respiratory fluoroquinolone
        - Either Zosyn, cefepime, imipenem, or meropenem, plus ciprofloxacin or levofloxacin
        - Either zosyn, cefepime, imipenem, or meropenem, plus amikacin or tobramycin, plus azithromycin
        - Either zosyn, cefepime, imipenem, or meropenem plus amikacin or tobramycin, plus levofloxacin or moxifloxacin
- MRSA:
    - Patients with exposure to nursing homes, receiving hemodialysis, or exposure to someone with skin and soft tissue infections
    - Add vancomycin or linezolid to current treatment

Etiology:

- Community acquired pneumonia:
    - Most common cause is **streptococcus pneumoniae**
    - Mycoplasma, chlamydia, viral (young and healthy)
    - Haemophilus influenza, Moraxella catarrhalis (COPD)
    - Legionella (smokers, elderly, immunocompromised, hotel/cruise)
    - Klebsiella and other gram negative rods (alcoholics, aspirators)
    - Staphylococcus aureus (post viral infection, IV drug abusers)
    - Influenza
    - Bordetella Pertussis (unvaccinated or adults with waning immunity)
    - Anthrax (bioterrorism)
    - Chlamydia psittaci (bird exposure)
    - Franciscella Tularensis (rabbit exposure)
    - Histoplasmosis (bird/bat droppings)
- Hospital acquired pneumonia:
    - Gram negative rods (pseudomonas, klebsiella, E. Coli, Enterobacter, serratia, Acinetobacter)
    - S. aureus, including MRSA
- Immunocompromised:
    - Legionella
    - PCP, fungi, nocardia, CMV, HSV
    - Non-TB mycobacteria

- Aspiration:
    - Chemical from gastric contents
    - Bacterial from oropharyngeal aspiration **(anaerobes)**

Risk Factors:

- Smoking
- Alcohol use
- Chronic comorbidities (COPD, CHF, neurologic diseases)
- PPI use long term

Pathogenesis:

- Hosts response to pathogens at the alveolar level damages the lung parenchyma
- Normal barriers are overcome (nares hairs, mucociliary clearance, gag reflex, cough, normal flora decreased)
- Alveolar macrophages clear pathogens, if this gets saturated, then pneumonia occurs
- **Hosts inflammation causes pneumonia (NOT the organism)**
- IL-1 and TNF alpha cause the fever
- Neutrophils extravasate into lung parenchyma, causes leukocytosis and purulent secretions
- RBC's can cross alveolar capillary membrane, causing hemoptysis
- Capillary leak causes infiltrate → rales, hypoxemia
- Initial phase- edema
- Red hepatization phase- erythrocytes plus neutrophils
- Grey hepatization phase- erythrocytes are lysed, neutrophils predominant with fibrin deposition, bacteria are gone
- Resolution phase- macrophages clear everything

Prevention:

- Pneumococcal vaccine
- Influenza vaccine annually
- Smoking cessation
- Education about stopping alcohol binge drinking

Complications:

- ARDS
- Pleural effusion
- MI
- CHF
- Acute renal failure
- COPD exacerbation
- Empyema
- Lung abscess
- Sepsis to septic shock
- DVT/PE

Admission Orders:

- Admit- floor (CURB-65 2), ICU (CURB-65 ≥ 3)
- Diagnosis- community acquired pneumonia
- Condition- stable
- Vital signs routine
- Allergies
- Activity as tolerated
- Nursing- supplemental O2 via NC to maintain O2 sat >92%
- Diet regular (if aspiration → NPO until evaluated)
- Fluids sepsis resuscitation
- Meds:
    o Ceftriaxone 1g Q24h plus azithromycin 500mg once, then 250mg
    o Acetaminophen 650mg PO Q6h prn pain/fever
- Labs/diagnostics:
    o CXR
    o Sputum gram stain and culture prior (if indicated) to antibiotics
    o Blood cultures x2 before antibiotics
    o BMP
    o CBC with differential
    o BNP
    o ABG
    o Urinary Ag for legionella and strep pneumonia if indicated
    o CRP
    o Procalcitonin

Discharge Information:

- Normal vital signs and normal mental status
- Tolerating PO antibiotics/fluids/food
- Safe home environment
- SaO2 ≥ 90% room air
- Pneumococcal vaccine and influenza vaccine before discharge if don't have them

Additional Notes:

- **Smoking cessation very important**
- Normal pulse with elevated temperature suggests atypical pneumonia

COPD

Definitions:

Chronic bronchitis- A clinical diagnosis: productive cough >3 months/year for ≥ 2 years

Emphysema- A pathological diagnosis: dilation/destruction of lung parenchyma

History:

In an outpatient setting, the diagnosis of COPD is usually a clinical suspicion in a person who has smoked for many years and has been having SOB with cough chronically. It would then be diagnosed with spirometry. In the inpatient setting, a COPD exacerbation occurs with either an increase in cough or sputum production, or increased dyspnea on exertion. History of prior exacerbations is important to know, as well as their baseline level of activity. It is also important to note that underlying 20% of COPD exacerbations is a pulmonary embolus, and that pneumonia occurs very commonly in exacerbations.

CC:

HPI:

- COLIDDERRS
    - *A patient with known lung disease who has increased sputum production, worsening dyspnea, wheezing, who is a smoker*
- Cough? Worsening?
- Sputum production and quality?
    - *Can help to see if they have a concurrent pneumonia*
- Increased DOE?
    - *Avoidance of exertion may be a first sign*
- Hx of exacerbations?
    - *What was done at the hospital?*
    - *History of intubations?*
    - *How long did it take to recover?*
    - *How is this same or different?*
- Baseline of activity?
    - *Worsening of activity from baseline level is a sign of exacerbation*
- Home oxygen use?
    - *Has oxygen requirement increased recently?*
- Fever/chills?
    - *Possible signs of co-existing pneumonia that needs treated*
- Ill contacts?
    - *Possible source of pneumonia or illness causing exacerbation*
- Nausea/vomiting?
    - *Tolerate PO meds or not*
- Diarrhea?
    - *Could be a sign of legionella, and possible volume depletion*
- Myalgias?
    - *Possible influenza, but also if pain needs to be addressed*
- Wheezing?
    - *Common symptom*

- Hemoptysis?
    - *Possible PE that needs to be ruled out*
- Chest pain?
    - *Possible PE or acute coronary syndrome that needs to be ruled out*
- Edema?
    - *Possible CHF as the cause*

ROS:

PMH:

- Hx of COPD?
    - *How severe?*
        - *Known PFT's?*
    - *Exacerbation history?*
    - *Home oxygen use?*
- Hx of CHF?
    - *Can mimic a COPD exacerbation of LHF*
- Hx of Asthma?
    - *Risk factor for COPD*
- Hx of Cystic fibrosis?
    - *Changes treatment and antibiotic coverage*
- Hx of A-fib?
    - *COPD a risk factor for A-fib and if they should be anticoagulated*
- Hx of Lung cancer?
    - *Radiation?*
    - *Pneumonitis?*
    - *Worsening symptoms?*
- Hx of Diabetes?
    - *Pseudomonas pneumonia and need to treat hyperglycemia*

Surgical H:

Social H:

- Alcohol, smoking, recreational drugs, job, living situation, sexual history

Family H:

- Hx of COPD?
- Hx of Heart disease?
- Hx of Asthma?

Allergies:

Medications:

- What medications they are taking and their compliance
- Home O2?

Physical Examination:

Vital signs, including O2 saturation, are important in case intubation is necessary. Altered mental status can be a sign of impending need for intubation. The classic 'blue bloaters' and 'pink puffers' are generally not seen, and is usually a combination of the two. Respiratory exam for obvious reasons is an important aspect of the exam.

- Vital signs
    - Tachypnea, tachycardia, O2 sats, BP
- General appearance
    - Accessory muscle use, cyanosis, pursed lips, tripod position, barrel chest, cachexia, cigarette odor
- Lymphadenopathy
- Oral mucosa for moist or dry
- Cardiac exam
    - JVD, S3 could indicate CHF, edema
- Respiratory exam
    - Hyper-resonance, prolonged expiratory phase (≥ 6 seconds), wheezing, barrel chest, accessory muscle use, tachypnea, paradoxical chest wall movement, decreased breath sounds
- Abdominal exam
    - Hepatomegaly could show RHF
- Dermatitis of hands from tripod position, nicotine stains
- Mental status exam
    - Part of CURB-65 if pneumonia present too

Differential Diagnosis:

- Pneumonia
    - *Could co-exist with COPD exacerbation*
- CHF
    - *LHF causes vascular congestion and can mimic COPD exacerbation, usually have more of a cardiac history*
- Asthma
    - *Usually a younger person with known diagnosis*
- Bronchiectasis
    - *Chronic cough, foul smelling sputum, recurrent or chronic pneumonia, hemoptysis*
- Cystic fibrosis
    - *Younger person with known diagnosis*
- **PE (20%)**
    - *Can be subtle, needs to be investigated*
- Pneumothorax
    - *Respiratory distress, asymmetric lung sounds, seen on CXR*
- Alpha-1 antitrypsin deficiency (younger person who doesn't smoke who has COPD symptoms classically)
- Pleural effusion
    - *Can be asymptomatic, but may present like any lung disease, then seen on CXR*
- Lung cancer

Labs:

- CBC with differential
    - Leukocytosis, look for polycythemia as secondary polycythemia may occur
- BMP
    - Look for any electrolyte abnormalities, and glucose as hyperglycemia needs to be treated
- BNP
    - Helps rule out CHF
- D-dimer if clinical suspicion for DVT
    - Use simplified Wells criteria to know high or low risk
- Troponins
    - Rule out MI causing pulmonary congestion
- ABG
    - Classic pattern is increased PCO2 with decreased PO2. In the acute setting get decreased pH, showing an acute respiratory acidosis. In chronic, have a respiratory acidosis with metabolic alkalosis as compensation (increased HCO3-)
- Sputum culture with gram stain
    - In case need specific antibiotics
- Procalcitonin
    - Can help with knowing if a bacterial infection is present as well and if antibiotics are needed

Imaging:

- EKG
    - Possible multifocal atrial tachycardia, A-fib, help rule out acute or chronic ischemia, PE pattern
- CXR
    - Hyperinflation, flattened diaphragm, enlarged retrosternal space
- Possibly CTA if high clinical suspicion for PE
    - Use simplified Wells criteria

Admittance/Staging and Prognosis:

- General floor admit:
    - **Anyone who the ED calls about, because if they are not at baseline after a couple of duoneb treatments then they need to be admitted**
    - Marked increase in baseline symptoms, outpatient treatment failure of an exacerbation, severe underlying COPD, change in mental status, significant comorbidities, poor home support, older age
- ICU admittance:
    - **Rising CO2 and need for BIPAP or intubation**
    - Change in mental status, severe dyspnea, poorly responsive to initial therapy, worsening hypoxemia (<40mmHg O2), severe hypercapnia (>60mmHg), severe acidosis (pH <7.25), mechanical ventilation, need for vasopressors
- BODE index:
    - **B**MI $\leq$21 (+1)

- Obstruction (fev1)- 50-64% (+1), 36-49% (+2), <35% (+3)
- **D**yspnea- walking (+1), after 100 yards (+2), with activities of daily living (+3)
- Exercise capacity (6 minute walk)- 250-349 meters (+1), 150-249 meters (+2), <149 meters (+3)
- 4 year survival 18% with 7-10 points
- mMRC (dyspnea assessment):
    - Grade 0- breathless with strenuous exercise
    - Grade 1- short of breath when hurrying on level ground or walking up a slight hill
    - Grade 2- on level ground, walk slower than people of the same age because of breathlessness, or have to stop for breath when walking at my own pace
    - Grade 3- stop for breath after walking about 100 yards or after a few minutes on level ground
    - Grade 4- too breathless to leave the house or breathless when driving
- Gold groups A-D
    - Group A- 0-1 exacerbations per year and no prior hospitalization for exacerbation with mMRC grade 0-1
    - Group B- 0-1 exacerbations per year and no prior hospitalization for exacerbation with mMRC grade $\geq$ 2
    - Group C- $\geq$ 2 exacerbations per year or $\geq$ 1 hospitalization for exacerbation with mMRC grade 0-1
    - Group D- $\geq$ 2 exacerbations per year or $\geq$ 1 hospitalization for exacerbations with mMRC grade $\geq$ 2

Treatment:

Acute Exacerbations:

- Supplemental O2 to keep SaO2 88-92%
- **Duoneb** - combines albuterol with ipratropium
    - **Main pharmacological treatment in exacerbation**
- Antibiotics if increased cough production:
    - Doxycycline or azithromycin
    - Amoxicillin, augmentin
    - Ceftriaxone
    - Levofloxacin, zosyn, or cefepime if you suspect pseudomonas could be present
- IV methylprednisolone Q6h 125mg or prednisolone 30-40mg QD for severe
    - **Steroids decrease length of stay**
    - **REDUCE trial (2013)-** A 5-day course of glucocorticoids is non-inferior to a 14-day course for treatment of acute COPD exacerbations in prevention of re-exacerbations at 180 days
- NIPPV if PaCO2 > 45mmHg, RR > 25
- Intubation if PaO2 < 55-60, increasing PaCO2, respiratory fatigue, change in mental status, hemodynamic instability
- Notice how there is **NOT Advair**, a long acting beta agonist and fluticasone, it is not warranted in acute exacerbations

Outpatient COPD Treatment:

- **Smoking cessation (most important, increases survival)**
    - Bupropion
    - Nicotine replacement
    - Varenecline
    - If a smoker quits, the rate of decline of FEV1 slows to that of someone of the same age who has never smoked. However, quitting does not result in complete reversal.
- Albuterol 2-4mg PO TID-QID or prn
- Ipratropium or tiotropium **(decreases number of hospitalizations)**
    - **UPLIFT trial (2008, NEJM)-** Tiotropium did not significantly slow the decline of FEV1, but did reduce the incidence of COPD exacerbations among individuals with moderate to severe COPD, and showed a trend towards improved survival
- Advair (fluticasone + salmeterol)
    - **TORCH trial (2007, NEJM)-** among patients with COPD, combination salmeterol/fluticasone therapy was associated with a reduction in the rate of COPD exacerbation and hospitalizations, but there was only a trend towards improved survival at 3 years (P=0.052)
- Indacaterol + glycopyrronium
    - **FLAME (COPD) trial (2016, NEJM)-** Among patients with COPD and mMRC dyspnea grade ≥ 2 symptoms, indacaterol + glycopyrronium (LABA + LAMA) is associated with a reduction in the annual rate of COPD exacerbations when compared to salmeterol + fluticasone (LABA + ICS)
- **Supplemental O2 (increases survival)**
    - Indications:
        - $SaO2 \leq 88\%$
        - $SaO2 \leq 90\%$ with pulmonary HTN or RHF
        - $HCT \geq 55\%$ + PaO2 55-59 mmHg
    - **NOTT trial (1980, Annals of Internal Medicine)-** In patients with COPD and hypoxemia, continuous oxygen therapy significantly reduces mortality when compared to nocturnal oxygen therapy
- **NOT** oral corticosteroids
- Can consider theophylline
- Pneumococcal vaccine
- Influenza vaccine
- Pulmonary rehab
- Lung volume reduction surgery/transplant
    - **NETT trial (2003, NEJM)-** Lung volume reduction surgery in patients with severe bilateral emphysema does not improve survival but is associated with improved exercise tolerance when compared to medical therapy alone. A survival benefit may be present for low- and moderate-risk patients with upper lobe emphysema and low exercise capacity.
- Azithromycin prophylaxis in the right setting
    - **Azithromycin for Prevention of Exacerbations of COPD (2011, NEJM)-** Among selected subjects with COPD, azithromycin taken daily for 1 year, when added to usual treatment, decreased the frequency of exacerbations and improved quality of life but caused hearing decrements in a small percentage of subjects. Although this

intervention could change microbial resistance patterns, the effect of this change is not known.

Etiology:

- **Smoking**
- Alpha-1 antitrypsin deficiency
- Chronic asthma
- Pathogens in acute exacerbation:
    - Streptococcus pneumoniae
    - H. influenza
    - Moraxella catarrhalis
    - Pseudomonas

Risk Factors:

- **Smoking**
- Alpha-1 Antitrypsin deficiency
- Occupational dusts (coal mining)
- Indoor air pollution and outdoor air pollution
- Impaired lung growth/development
- Recurrent infections
- Second hand smoke

Pathogenesis:

- Airflow limitation and **air trapping**
- Hyperplasia, mucus, fibrosis
- Parenchymal inflammation and fibrosis
- Elastase > anti-elastase
- Oxidants from smoke, macrophages get activated, proteinases and chemokines produced, inflammatory cells come in
- Loss of cilia
- Large airways get goblet cell hyperplasia causing cough/sputum, also smooth muscle hypertrophy and bronchial hyper-reactivity
- Small airways get loss of clara cells, decreased surfactant → increased surface tension → airway narrowing and collapse with fibrosis
- Lung parenchyma gets destroyed/fibrosed in emphysema, get a decreased diffusion capacity → decreased gas exchange
    - Centriacinar (smoking) → upper lungs
    - Panacinar (alpha-1 antitrypsin deficiency) → lower lobes
- **FEV1/FVC ratio decreases (<80%)**
- Hyperinflation from air trapping
- **V/Q mismatch, NOT shunting**

Complications:

- Respiratory failure
- Pulmonary HTN
- Cor pulmonale
- Cachexia/weakness

- Anemia
- CAD
- CHF
- Depression
- Infections
- Disability
- Lung cancer
- A-fib
- Multi-focal atrial tachycardia
- Secondary polycythemia

Admission Orders:

- Admit to floor or ICU
- Diagnosis COPD exacerbation
- Condition stable, guarded, critical
- Vital signs ICU routine or routine
- Allergies
- Activity as tolerated
- Nursing O2 to maintain SaO2 of 88-92%
- Diet regular
- Fluids
- Meds:
    - IV methylprednisolone 125mg IV
    - Duoneb Q4h
    - Antibiotics
        - Amoxicillin, augmentin
        - Ceftriaxone
        - Levofloxacin, zosyn, or cefepime if suspect pseudomonas could be present
    - Nicotine patch 21mg QD
- Labs/diagnostics:
    - CBC with differential
    - BMP
    - Sputum, blood, urine cultures
    - BNP
    - Troponins
    - ABG
    - EKG
    - CXR
    - D-dimer if indicated
    - CTA if indicated
    - Procalcitonin

Discharge Information:

- Assess for home O2 needs (see above)
- Education of outpatient meds (MDI education)
- Smoking cessation education
- Follow up with PCP
- Pulmonary consult if age <40, ≥ 2 episodes/year, rapidly worsening disease, severe disease (FEV1 < 50%), need for home O2

Additional Notes:

- Important clinical trials:
    - **REDUCE trial (2013, NEJM)-** A 5-day course of glucocorticoids is non-inferior to a 14-day course for treatment of acute COPD exacerbations in prevention of re-exacerbations at 180 days
    - **UPLIFT trial (2008, NEJM)-** Tiotropium did not significantly slow the decline of FEV1, but did reduce the incidence of COPD exacerbations among individuals with moderate to severe COPD, and showed a trend towards improved survival
    - **TORCH trial (2007, NEJM)-** among patients with COPD, combination salmeterol/fluticasone therapy was associated with a reduction in the rate of COPD exacerbation and hospitalizations, but there was only a trend towards improved survival at 3 years (P=0.052)
    - **FLAME (COPD) trial (2016, NEJM)-** Among patients with COPD and mMRC dyspnea grade ≥ 2 symptoms, indacaterol + glycopyrronium (LABA + LAMA) is associated with a reduction in the annual rate of COPD exacerbations when compared to salmeterol + fluticasone (LABA + ICS)
    - **NOTT trial (1980, Annals of Internal Medicine)-** In patients with COPD and hypoxemia, continuous oxygen therapy significantly reduces mortality when compared to nocturnal oxygen therapy
    - **NETT trial (2003, NEJM)-** Lung volume reduction surgery in patients with severe bilateral emphysema does not improve survival but is associated with improved exercise tolerance when compared to medical therapy alone. A survival benefit may be present for low- and moderate-risk patients with upper lobe emphysema and low exercise capacity.
    - **Azithromycin for Prevention of Exacerbations of COPD (2011, NEJM)-** Among selected subjects with COPD, azithromycin taken daily for 1 year, when added to usual treatment, decreased the frequency of exacerbations and improved quality of life but caused hearing decrements in a small percentage of subjects. Although this intervention could change microbial resistance patterns, the effect of this change is not known.

Asthma

Definitions:

<u>Asthma-</u> A chronic inflammatory disorder with airway hyperresponsiveness plus variable airflow obstruction

History:

When determining if someone has asthma, the history is used to determine whether the person actually has asthma, or if there is some other reason for their chronic or intermittent cough. If the person has known asthma and is presenting to the hospital, then it is important to inquire about a history of exacerbations, medications they take, how often they take those medications, and if they are actually compliant with their medications.

CC:

HPI:

- COLIDDERRS
    - *Patient with SOB, wheezing, hyperresonant lung fiends, with prolonged expiratory phase, and exposure to a trigger (cold air, allergens), and CBC with eosinophilia and nasal polyps on exam*
- Symptoms like this before, and if so, intermittent?
- Chest tightness?
- Wheezing?
    - *Most common symptom*
- Dyspnea?
    - *Worsening?*
- Relief with rescue inhalers?
    - *If so, as much relief as usual? Or not as much?*
- Baseline asthma status?
    - Albuterol use per day/week
    - Nighttime use of albuterol?
    - Other asthma meds?
- Allergies?
    - *Can be the cause of asthma, or can cause an asthma exacerbation because of inflammation*
- Prior exacerbations and outcomes?
    - *Will help you know whether you need to admit the patient, and where they need to go (ie floor, ICU)*
    - *Ask about prior intubations, history of labile asthma, frequent hospitalizations, ED visit in the past 12 months for asthma, low adherence to inhaled steroids*
- Change in mental status?
    - *May be a reason to need intubation or admit to the ICU*
- Recent illness?
    - *Can be a cause of asthma exacerbation, or may be a pneumonia, bronchitis, URI, etc*
- Precipitants?

47

- *Pollens, house dust, molds, cockroaches, cats, dogs, cold air, viral infections, tobacco smoke, medications (beta blockers, aspirin), and exercise*

ROS:

PMH:

- Hx of COPD/restrictive lung diseases?
    - *May be the reason for the SOB and wheezing*
- Hx of Allergies?
    - *May be the cause of an asthma exacerbation, or may have exacerbated it by inflammation*
- Hx of Cystic fibrosis?
    - *Will usually have the diagnosis already*

Surgical H:

Social H:

- Alcohol, smoking, recreational drugs, job, living situation, sexual history

Family H:

Allergies:

Medications:

- Compliance with meds? Using more of rescue inhaler?
- Beta blockers?
- Aspirin?

Physical Examination:

The physical exam in an asthma exacerbation is focused on the severity of respiratory distress the person is experiencing. Mental status is important, as well as signs of respiratory fatigue that could be signs of impending respiratory failure.

- Vital signs
    - RR, HR, BP, O2 sats, temp
- Lymphadenopathy
    - May show that it is an infectious process rather than just asthma
- Oral mucosa for moisture, dry, or pharyngeal erythema
    - Pharyngeal erythema may show asthma or GERD as the cause of wheezing
- Nasal polyps
    - Cystic fibrosis may be the cause, or aspirin induced asthma
- Cardiac
    - Pulsus paradoxus may be present (>10mmHg drop in BP with inspiration)
    - JVD
- Respiratory

- Wheezing is a classic sign, decreased breath sounds can be a sign of increased severity. Percussion could show hyperresonance.
  - Accessory muscle use
  - Use of full sentences or not
  - Look for tracheal deviation and asymmetric breath sounds which could be tension pneumothorax
- Signs of skin atopic dermatitis
  - Classic finding in atopic asthma
- Cyanosis
- Mental status

Differential Diagnosis:

- COPD
  - *Usually older, chronic cough and SOB, smoker, asthma is a risk factor to get COPD*
- Pneumonia
  - *Sudden onset of chills, fever, productive cough (rather than dry), myalgias, will have CXR findings*
- Pneumothorax
  - *Asymmetric breath sounds, tracheal deviation*
- PE
  - *May have hemoptysis, but can present just like asthma and needs to be investigated*
- Panic attack
  - *Usually has no previous diagnosis of asthma, and has some sort of emotional fear or psychiatric history*
- CHF
  - *Due to edema of airways and congestion of bronchial mucosa can cause wheezing, usually is older and has a cardiac history and will have edema*
- GERD
  - *Older person who has history of reflux pain after meals, and may get wheezing*
- Bronchiectasis
  - *Chronic cough, foul smelling, recurrent or chronic pneumonias, possible hemoptysis*
- Allergic bronchopulmonary aspergillus
  - *Will be more infectious setting than asthma exacerbation, but is an allergic reaction that causes wheezing*
- Cystic fibrosis
  - *Usually has a diagnosis of it already*
- Eosinophilic pneumonia
  - *Cough, fever, increasing breathlessness, and night sweats, occurs quickly*
- Bronchiolitis obliterans
  - *Shortness of breath and dry cough, usually will have a normal peak expiratory flow*
- Foreign body aspiration
  - *Usually was seen or part of history*
- Vocal cord paralysis/dysfunction
  - *Can cause wheezing but can have no SOB, and usually change in speech*

- Laryngotracheal mass
    - *Usually has stridor*
- Tracheal stenosis
    - *Gradually worsening dyspnea particularly DOE, and usually is stridor, which can be mistaken for wheezing*
- Tracheomalacia
    - *Usually has stridor*
- Angioedema
    - *Throat swelling, possible ACEI use*

Labs:

- ABG if severe
    - Hypocarbia is common as the patient is tachypneic, hypoxemia may be present
    - If CO2 levels start to increase or go back to normal, may be sign of impending respiratory failure and necessity for intubation
- CBC with differential
    - May show elevated eosinophils, look for leukocytosis as it may show infectious process present
- CMP
    - Look for electrolyte abnormalities
- Possible D-dimer
    - Use simplified Wells criteria
- Sputum culture
    - May be an infectious process
- Blood culture
    - May be an infectious process

Imaging:

- **Peak expiratory flow**
    - Do this at beginning of ER visit, and then intermittently throughout hospital stay
    - Normal: 450-650 L/min (men), 350-500 L/min (women)
    - Mild: >300 L/min
    - Moderate to severe: 100-300 L/min
    - Severe: <100 L/min
- CXR
    - Not always required, but will usually be done in any case of SOB
    - May show hyperinflation in severe asthma, normal in non-severe
    - Do to exclude other conditions (pneumonia, pneumothorax, pneumomediastinum, foreign body aspiration)
- **PFT's are required for diagnosis**, usually done in outpatient setting
    - Decreased FEV1, decreased FVC, decreased FEV1/FVC ratio
    - Increase in FEV1 > 12% with albuterol
    - Decrease in FEV1 >20% with methacholine or histamine
    - Increase in diffusion capacity of lung for CO

Admission:

Floor Admission:

- History of labile asthma
- Frequent hospitalizations
- ED visit in past 12 months for asthma
- Low adherence to inhaled steroids

ICU Admittance:

- Status asthmaticus
- Prior intubations
- Peak expiratory flow <30% of predicted improving <10% with treatment
- Signs of impending respiratory failure:
    - Change in mental status
    - Worsening fatigue
    - PCO_2 >42

Treatment:

Treatment of Acute Asthma Exacerbation:

- Supplemental O2 by mask to maintain SaO_2 >90%
- Albuterol nebulizer 2.5-5mg Q20 min
    - **Mainstay of treatment**
- Methylprednisolone 125mg IV now, then prednisone 0.5-1 mg/kg PO after
    - If ICU, only do methylprednisolone 125mg Q6h
- Ipratropium Nebulizer 0.5mg Q20 min if severe
    - **Duoneb** to combine albuterol and ipratropium
- $MgSO_2$ 2g IV over 20 min if severe $\pm$ heliox
- Antibiotics if severe exacerbation or suspicion of infection
- Intubation for respiratory failure

```
Reassessment after 1-3h of Tx
```

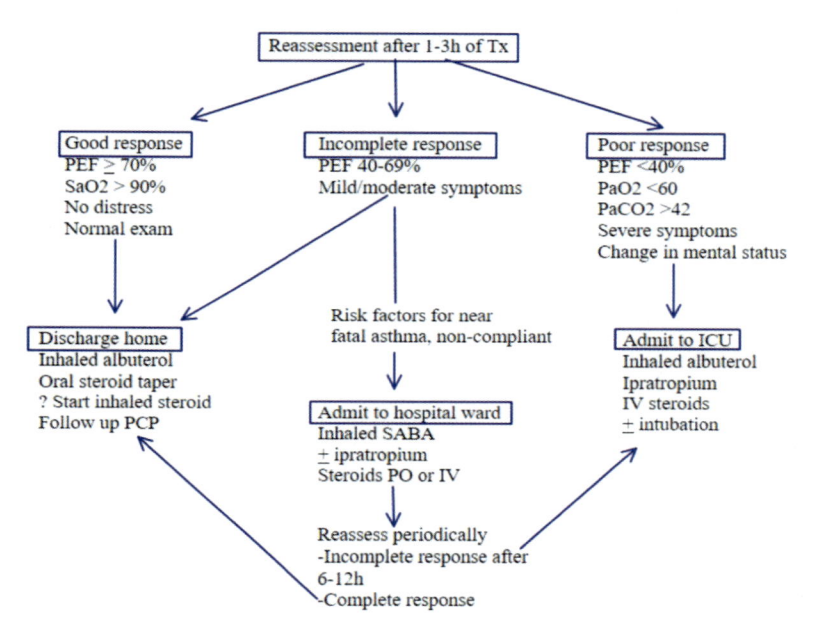

- **Good response**
  - PEF ≥ 70%
  - SaO2 > 90%
  - No distress
  - Normal exam
  - → **Discharge home**
    - Inhaled albuterol
    - Oral steroid taper
    - ? Start inhaled steroid
    - Follow up PCP

- **Incomplete response**
  - PEF 40-69%
  - Mild/moderate symptoms
  - Risk factors for near fatal asthma, non-compliant
  - → **Admit to hospital ward**
    - Inhaled SABA
    - ± ipratropium
    - Steroids PO or IV
  - Reassess periodically
    - Incomplete response after 6-12h
    - Complete response

- **Poor response**
  - PEF <40%
  - PaO2 <60
  - PaCO2 >42
  - Severe symptoms
  - Change in mental status
  - → **Admit to ICU**
    - Inhaled albuterol
    - Ipratropium
    - IV steroids
    - ± intubation

Treatment of Chronic Asthma/Prevention:

- Stepwise approach:
    - <u>Mild intermittent</u>- symptoms two or fewer times per week but <2 times a month at night
        - Albuterol prn
    - <u>Mild persistent</u>- symptoms 2 or more times per week but not everyday but 3-4 times a month at night
        - Add fluticasone (flovent)
        - Do NOT add a long acting beta agonist prior to an ICS
        - **SMART trial (2006, Chest)-** Salmeterol increases the risk of respiratory-related deaths, particularly among African American patient and those not using an inhaled corticosteroid
    - <u>Moderate persistent</u>- daily symptoms; frequent exacerbations but >1 times a week at night
        - Replace flovent with Advair (salmeterol + fluticasone) in addition to keeping albuterol
    - <u>Severe persistent</u>- continual symptoms, frequent exacerbations and often 7 times/week
        - Albuterol + higher dose of advair
    - <u>Very severe persistent</u>-
        - Add prednisone 7.5-60mg PO

				OCS
			LABA	LABA
		LABA	ICS High dose	ICS High dose
	ICS Low dose	ICS Low dose		
Short-acting β_2-agonist as required for symptom relief				
Mild intermittent	Mild persistent	Moderate persistent	Severe persistent	Very severe persistent

- Add on meds:
    - Antileukotrienes- monteleukast 10mg PO QPM
    - Cromones- Cromolyn sodium 200mg PO QID or Nedocromil
    - Theophylline 300-600mg/day PO
    - Anti-IgE- Omalizumab (Xolair) 150-375 subQ Q2-4 weeks
        - Expensive, IgE must be in a specific range
    - Immunotherapy
    - Avoid triggers- allergies, exercise, fog, cold weather
- Influenza vaccine
- Avoid sedatives

Etiology:

- Genetic and environmental factors

Risk Factors:

- Endogenous factors- genetics, atopy, airway hyperresonpsiveness, gender, ethnicity, obesity, early viral infections
- Environmental factors- indoor allergens (pets, dust mites), outdoor pollens (pollen), occupational sensitizers, passive smoking, respiratory infections, diet, acetaminophen
- Triggers- allergens, upper respiratory infections, exercise and hyperventilation, cold air, sulfur dioxide, irritant gases, beta-blockers, ASA, stress, GERD, hormones (pre-menstrual asthma)

Pathogenesis:

- **Triad:**
    - Airway inflammation
    - Airway hyperresponsiveness
    - Reversible airflow obstruction
- **Inflammatory process**
- Airway mucosa is infiltrated with activated eosinophils and T-lymphocytes with activation of mast cells
- Epithelium often sheds → thickened airway and edematous airway
- Mucous plug from goblet cells
- Vasodilation and angiogenesis
- Narrowing of airways, with inflammation of mucosa from trachea to terminal bronchioles, mainly bronchi

- **Local IgE production**
- **Mast cells activated by allergens through an IgE dependent mechanism** and binding of specific IgE to mast cells
- Macrophages activated, cytokines are released, dendritic cells activated, TH2 cells release IL-2 and TNF alpha
- **Eosinophils** cause release of free radicals → inflammation
- Nitric oxide released → vasodilation
- Epithelial shedding, fibrosis of basement membrane (III/IV collagen)
- Smooth muscle hypertrophy/hyperplasia
- Mucous hypersecretion from submucosal gland hyperplasia

Complications:

- Symptoms inferring with activities of daily living
- Permanent narrowing of bronchial tubes
- EM visits and hospitalizations
- Side effects from medications
- COPD
- Death

Admission Orders:

- Admit to floor or ICU
- Diagnosis asthma exacerbation
- Condition stable, guarded, or critical
- Vital signs routine or ICU routine
- Allergies
- Activity as tolerated
- Nursing check peak expiratory flow QD and educate patient in performing at home, O2 maintain >90%
- Diet regular
- Fluids
- Meds:
    - Methylprednisolone 125mg IV now, prednisone 60mg QD
    - Albuterol nebulizer Q4h or Q1h prn SOB/wheezing
    - Ipratropium nebulizer Q4h
    - Or **Duoneb**
- Labs/diagnostics:
    - ABG
    - CBC
    - CMP
    - CXR
    - Sputum culture
    - Blood cultures

Discharge Information:

- Ensure adequate meds are prescribed with education of how to use them
- Use stepwise approach to decide what medications to give
- Provide a peak expiratory flow monitor
- Educate on triggers, smoking cessation

- Follow up in 7 days with PCP or asthma specialist if it was life threatening

Additional Notes:

- Important clinical trials:
    - **SMART trial (2006, Chest)-** Salmeterol increases the risk of respiratory-related deaths, particularly among African American patient and those not using an inhaled corticosteroid

Pleural Effusion

Definitions:

Lights Criteria- helps determine whether the effusion is transudative or exudative. To be exudative, any of the following three criteria must be met:

1. Pleural fluid:serum protein >0.5
2. Pleural fluid:serum LDH > 0.6
3. Pleural fluid LDH >2/3 upper normal serum limit (~200)

History:

Usually a pleural effusion is a part of another clinical entity. It will usually be seen on CXR and CT when lung disease is suspected or if physical exam supports it being present. It is often asymptomatic.

CC:

HPI:

- COLIDDERRS
    - *Exertional dyspnea with pleural effusion found on X-ray*
- Dyspnea on exertion?
    - *Most common symptom*
- Trauma?
    - *Can cause chylothorax, hemothorax, etc.*
- COPD history?
    - *Another cause of DOE*
- Any respiratory disease history?
- Malignancy history?
    - *Common cause of chylothorax*
- TB history?
    - *Common cause of exudative process*
- Recent illness?
    - *Viral and bacterial processes can cause pleural effusion*
- Cough?
    - *Common symptom*
- Orthopnea?
    - *CHF is the most common cause of pleural effusion*
- Edema?
    - *CHF is the most common cause of pleural effusion, but also nephrotic syndrome or cirrhosis*
- CHF history?
    - *Number one cause of pleural effusions*
- Paroxysmal nocturnal dyspnea?
    - *CHF is the most common cause of pleural effusion*

ROS:

PMH:

- Hx of COPD?
    - *Can cause SOB, more susceptible to pleural effusions*
- Hx of Respiratory disease?
    - *More susceptible to pleural effusions*
- Hx of Malignancy?
    - *Can lead to chylothorax or malignant pleural effusion*
- Hx of TB?
    - *Can lead to exudative pleural effusions*
- Hx of CHF?
    - *Most common cause of pleural effusions, transudative*

Surgical H:

- Recent thoracic or abdominal surgery?

Social H:

- Alcohol, smoking, recreational drugs, job, living situation, sexual history

Family H:

Allergies:

Medications:

Physical Examination:

The physical exam is usually not a big part of diagnosing a pleural effusion, it will just help support a clinical suspicion of findings on imaging.

- Vital signs
    - Tachypnea, fever, O2 sats
- Respiratory
    - Dullness to percussion, crackles, decreased tactile fremitus, decreased breath sounds over the effusion
- Edema
    - Looking for signs of CHF, cirrhosis, nephrotic syndrome

Differential Diagnosis:

- Atelectasis
    - *SOB, can be with chronic lung disease, will be seen differently on CXR*
- Chronic pleural thickening
    - *Chronic lung disease, pleural cancer*
- Lobar consolidation
    - *Pneumonia*
- Subdiaphragmatic process
    - *Cirrhosis, nephrotic syndrome*
- Pneumonia
- PE
    - *Always needs to be ruled out with SOB, use simplified Wells criteria*

Labs:

- Get pleural fluid total protein, LDH, and if indicated, glucose, cytology, differential cell count, culture, gram stain, pH and markers for TB (see below for indications to order those from pleural fluid)
    - **Four C's from pleural fluid:**
        - Chemistry (glucose, protein)
        - Cytology
        - Cell count (CBC with diff)
        - Culture
- Need serum LDH and protein for Lights criteria
- CBC with differential
    - Look for leukocytosis
- CMP
    - Look for liver function tests, electrolyte imbalances suggesting kidney disease
- PF NT-proBNP
    - > 1500 pg/ml → CHF effusion

Imaging:

- CXR PA/lateral and lateral decubitus (need 250ml to show up)
    - Blunting of costophrenic angle
- Chest ultrasound
- Thoracentesis if loculated
- Thoracostomy if loculated
- Thoracotomy if empyema
- CT possibly after thoracentesis

Diagnostic Algorithm:

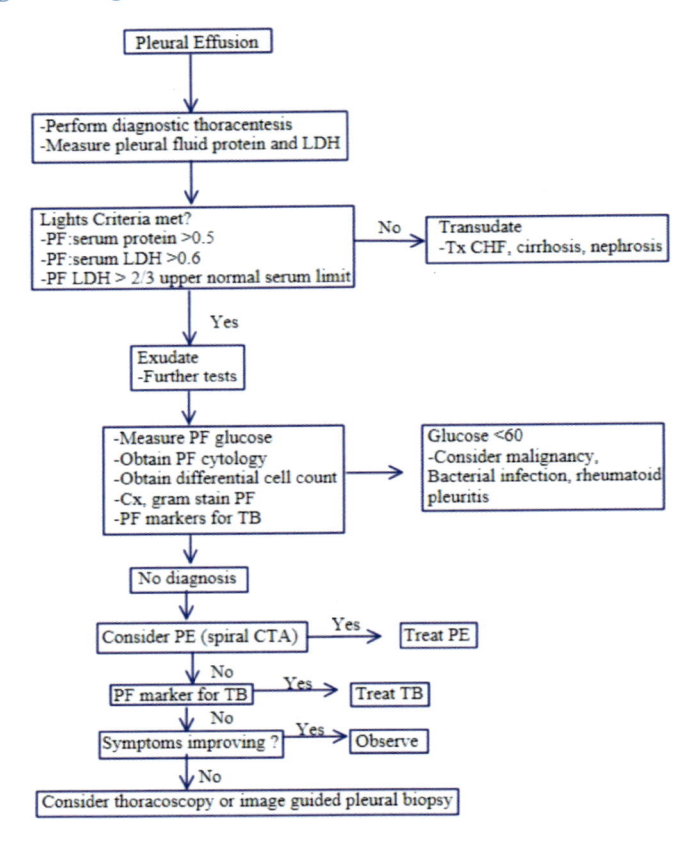

```
Pleural Effusion
      │
      ▼
-Perform diagnostic thoracentesis
-Measure pleural fluid protein and LDH
      │
      ▼
Lights Criteria met?                    No     Transudate
-PF:serum protein >0.5              ─────────▶ -Tx CHF, cirrhosis, nephrosis
-PF:serum LDH >0.6
-PF LDH > 2/3 upper normal serum limit
      │ Yes
      ▼
Exudate
-Further tests
      │
      ▼
-Measure PF glucose                         Glucose <60
-Obtain PF cytology                         -Consider malignancy,
-Obtain differential cell count      ────▶  Bacterial infection, rheumatoid
-Cx, gram stain PF                          pleuritis
-PF markers for TB
      │
      ▼
No diagnosis
      │
      ▼
Consider PE (spiral CTA) ──Yes──▶ Treat PE
      │ No
      ▼
PF marker for TB ──Yes──▶ Treat TB
      │ No
      ▼
Symptoms improving? ──Yes──▶ Observe
      │ No
      ▼
Consider thoracoscopy or image guided pleural biopsy
```

Indications for Thoracentesis:

- Any new unexplained pleural effusion
- All effusions >1cm in decubitus view of CXR
    - Can help diagnose and can be therapeutic
- Asymmetry of effusion
    - More likely to be from trauma or an infectious process if bilateral
- Fever
    - More likely to be an infectious process
- Failure to resolve despite treatment of what the underlying cause was

Etiologies and their Treatment:

- **Transudates:**
    - CHF
    - Cirrhosis

- o PE
- o Nephrotic syndrome
- o Peritoneal dialysis
- o Hypoalbuminemia
- o Atelectasis
- **Exudates:**
    - o Bacterial pneumonia, tuberculosis
    - o Malignancy, metastatic disease
    - o Viral infection
    - o PE
    - o Collagen vascular disease
- CHF:
    - o **Most common cause of pleural effusion**
    - o Perform thoracentesis if effusions are not bilateral and comparable in size, febrile, or pleuritic chest pain
    - o Otherwise treat CHF with diuresis
    - o PF NT-proBNP > 1500 pg/ml → CHF effusion
- Hepatic hydrothorax:
    - o Ascites from cirrhosis
    - o Treat the cirrhosis/ascites
- Parapneumonic effusion:
    - o Bacterial pneumonia, lung abscess, bronchiectasis, empyema
    - o Acute febrile illness, fever, chest pain, sputum, weight loss, leukocytosis
    - o If free fluid separates the lung from the chest wall by >10mm → therapeutic thoracentesis **(drain <1.5L to avoid re-expansion pulmonary edema)**
    - o Indications for more invasive procedures:
        - Loculated PF
        - PF glucose <60mg/dl
        - pH <7.2 of pleural fluid
        - + gram stain or culture
        - Gross pus in pleural space
    - o Consider chest tube with tpA 10mg and deoxyribonuclease 5mg or thoracoscopy with breakdown of adhesions
    - o Need anaerobic antibiotic coverage, usually start with zosyn
- Effusion secondary to malignancy:
    - o ~75% from lung, breast carcinoma, and lymphoma
    - o Dyspnea with **exudate and decreased glucose**
    - o Diagnosis is by cytology, **if initially negative, do another thoracentesis for more cytology** (increases the sensitivity), do thoracoscopy next if malignancy strongly considered, do pleural abrasion
    - o Alternative is CT/US needle biopsy
    - o Treat symptomatically, if dyspnea relieved with therapeutic thoracentesis, can 1) insert small indwelling catheter, 2) tube thoracostomy with doxycycline (500mg)
- Mesothelioma:
    - o Primary tumor, usually related to **asbestos** exposure (even though bronchogenic carcinoma is more common with asbestos exposure)
    - o Chest pain with SOB, pleural thickening, shrunken hemithorax
    - o Diagnosed with image guidance needle biopsy or thorascopy
- Effusion secondary to PE:
    - o **Overlooked** diagnosis when pleural effusion is present

- Dyspnea is most common symptom
- Usually an exudate
- Spiral CTA or V/Q scan
- Treat the PE
- TB:
    - Relatively uncommon in the US
    - Fever, weight loss, dyspnea, pleuritic chest pain
    - **Exudate with small lymphocytes and + Adenosine deaminase/interferon γ**
    - Treat the TB
- Effusion due to virus:
    - Don't be too aggressive with treatment, especially if improving
- Chylothorax:
    - Thoracic duct disrupted
    - Most commonly from trauma (surgery), or from mediastinal tumors
    - Thoracentesis produces **milky fluid**
    - **Triglycerides in thoracentesis are > 110mg/dl**
    - Treatment of choice is chest tube + octreotide
    - Can do ligation of thoracic duct or shunt
- Hemothorax:
    - Bloody pleural fluid, trauma, ruptured blood vessel, tumor
    - Tube thoracostomy or repair of pleura
    - If hemorrhage exceeds 200ml/hr → thoracoscopy or thoracotomy
- Other causes:
    - Esophageal rupture (increased amylase)
    - Pancreatic disease (increased amylase)
    - Intraabdominal abscess
    - Meigs syndrome
    - Drugs (eosinophilic)
    - Bypass
    - Nephrosis
    - Peritoneal dialysis
    - SVC obstruction
    - Myxedema
    - Urinothorax (Cr in pleural fluid)
    - Diaphragmatic hernia
    - SLE
    - Sjogrens
    - Wegeners
    - Chrug-strauss
    - Sarcoidosis
    - Uremia
    - Radiation
    - Iatrogenic

Pathogenesis:

- Pleural fluid formation exceeds pleural fluid absorption
- Either excess fluid formation (from interstitial spaces of lung, parietal pleura, or peritoneal cavity), or decreased fluid removal from lymphatics
- Transudate:
    - Increased capillary pressure (CHF) or decreased plasma oncotic pressure (hypoalbuminemia, like in cirrhosis or nephrotic syndrome)

- Exudate:
  - Increased permeability of pleural surfaces or decreased lymphatic flow

Additional Notes:

-

Venous Thromboembolism (PE/DVT)

Definitions:

<u>Low risk PE:</u> PE is present but no RV strain, increased troponin, increased BNP, or hypotension

<u>Submassive PE:</u> PE is present with RV strain, increased troponin, increased BNP, but no hypotension

<u>Massive PE:</u> PE is present with above signs with hypotension or cardiogenic shock

<u>Provoked DVT:</u> DVT in the setting of either active cancer/treatment of cancer in the last 6 months, recent immobilization, or major surgery

History:

The presentation of DVT and PE's can be subtle, and easily missed if the healthcare provider does not have a clinical suspicion. This can be a life threatening process, deeming it necessary to be ruled out in many clinical situations. It is important to know and ask about risk factors for VTE, which are listed below in the risk factors section.

CC: May be nothing. May be SOB/DOE, racing HR, swollen painful calf, cough, hemoptysis, etc.

HPI:

- COLIDDERRS
    - *A patient with SOB, hemoptysis, pleuritic chest pain, tachycardia, tachypnea, hypoxia, hypocapnia, unilateral leg swelling that is painful and erythematous who has been immobile and has cancer or recent surgery*
- PE:
    - SOB?
        - *Present in 73% of PE's*
    - Pleuritic chest pain?
        - *Present in 66% of PE's*
    - Cough?
        - *Present in 37% of PE's*
    - Hemoptysis?
        - *Present in 13% of PE's*
    - DOE?
    - Palpitations?
    - Syncope?
        - **PESIT trial (2016, NEJM)-** In patients admitted for first episode of syncope, 17% were found to have PE after a standardized, guideline-based inpatient evaluation. PE was identified in 12.7% of patients with an alternative etiology for syncope and 25.4% of patients who did not. PE was identified in 25% of patients without typical signs or symptoms.
- DVT:

- Leg swelling/pain?
  - *Worse with dependency/walking, better with elevation/rest*
- Recent long travel or immobilization?
- Recent major surgery?
- Active cancer/treatment of cancer in last 6 months?
- F/c?
- Pregnant?

ROS:

PMH:

- Hx of CHF?
  - *Can have lower extremity swelling mimicking DVT, or tachypnea/SOB mimicking PE*
- Hx of Cancer?
  - *Makes you in a hypercoagulable state*
- Hx of COPD?
  - *Can mimic PE symptoms*
- Hx of CKD?
  - *Makes you in a hypercoagulable state plus adds edema*
- Hx of SLE?
  - *Makes you in a hypercoagulable state possibly*

Surgical H:

- Any recent surgery
  - *Especially orthopedic surgery of long bones/pelvis which can lead to fat embolus PE*

Social H:

- Alcohol, smoking, recreational drugs, job, living situation, sexual history
  - *Smoking makes you more hypercoagulable*

Family H:

- Hx of blood clots?
  - *History of blood clots in family can lead you to investigate genetic causes of clots (ie factor V Leiden mutation, prothrombin mutation, etc.)*

Allergies:

Medications:

- Birth control?
  - *Increased estrogen state is hypercoagulable*
- Hormone therapy (estrogen)?
  - *Increased estrogen state is hypercoagulable*
- On anticoagulation (warfarin, xarelto, eliquis, etc.)?

o   *If on anticoagulation and still clotting then need further intervention*

Physical Examination:

Vital signs can range from normal to very abnormal. A full lung exam and exam for LE pain/swelling is important. It is important to note for JVD which could symbolize a very large pulmonary embolus. Cyanosis may be present.

- Vital signs
    - o   Tachypnea (70% of PE's) is the most common sign/symptom of PE, tachycardia (30% of PE's), hypoxemia, even fever can be present
        - **If tachycardia and suspecting PE, make them walk with pulse ox on**, if their sats drop, they may have a PE, if it doesn't, lower chance they do
    - o   Hypotension may be a sign of massive pulmonary embolus
- Full lung exam
    - o   Rales (51% of PE's)
- Cardiac
    - o   S4 (24% of PE's)
    - o   Loud P2 may be present (23% of PE's)
    - o   JVD
- Edema
- Leg pain/swelling/palpable cord
    - o   Homan's sign
- Venous stasis

Differential Diagnosis:

- PE:
    - o   MI
        - *Can lead to SOB, tachypnea, and edema*
    - o   Pneumonia
        - *Fever, SOB, tachypnea, productive cough, pleuritic chest pain*
    - o   Pericarditis
        - *Pleuritic chest pain, pain better with leaning forward, pain radiating to trapezius ridge, friction rub, diffuse ST segment elevation and PR segment depression*
    - o   CHF
        - *SOB from vascular congestion (LHF), edema*
    - o   Pleuritis
        - *Long time smoker or lung disease, just cough or pleuritic chest pain*
    - o   Pneumothorax
        - *Respiratory distress, asymmetric breath sounds*
    - o   Pericardial tamponade
        - *Hypotension, JVD, decreased heart sounds (Becks triad), pulsus paradoxus, narrowed pulse pressure*
- DVT:
    - o   Muscular strain
        - *Some sort of trauma or exercise induced pain, bruising*
    - o   Bakers cyst

- Felt on physical exam, US shows the cyst
- Achilles tendon rupture
  - Positive Thompson's test, unable to plantarflex the foot
- Cellulitis
  - Have signs of fever, some sort of wound, warm feeling, no clot on US
- Superficial thrombophlebitis
  - More superficial and more along veins
- Lymphatic obstruction (ie pelvic tumor)
  - More edema of the entire leg
- Reflex sympathetic dystrophy
  - Swelling, redness with vasomotor instability, hyperhidrosis, coolness to the touch

Labs:

- CBC
  - Look for polycythemia, anemia, thrombocytosis, leukocytosis
- CMP
- D-dimer
  - Use this to rule out DVT/PE in low clinical situations (see simplified Wells criteria below)
- BNP
  - Can see if CHF may be the cause of the SOB, tachypnea, edema, etc.
- Troponins
  - If patient has chest pain, SOB, edema, etc.
- Hypercoagulable panel
  - Don't do this very often, and not suggested to test for unless very certain circumstances
  - APC Resistance, Antithrombin III Activity, Factor V(Leiden) Mutation Analysis w/ Reflex to HR2*, Protein C Activity, Protein C Antigen, Protein S Antigen, Free, dRVVT Screen w/Reflex to dRVVT Confirm & dRVVT 1:1 Mix, PTT-LA w/Reflex to Hexagonal Phase Confirmation, Homocysteine (Cardiovascular), Cardiolipin Antibody (IgG), Cardiolipin Antibody (IgM)
- ABG depending on level of respiratory distress

Imaging:

- EKG:
  - **Most common finding is sinus tachycardia**
  - S1Q3T3, acute right bundle branch block, right axis deviation, and RV strain (ST depression in II and T wave inversion in anterior precordial leads (V1-4)) are other patterns
  - Also are looking for signs of ischemia, ventricular hypertrophy, pericarditis, etc.
- CXR:
  - Westermarks sign, Hamptons Hump, Palla's sign
  - **Someone with normal CXR and hypoxemia, consider PE**
  - Also looking for any signs of infection, cardiomegaly, etc.
- Venous Doppler:

- Initial test for DVT
- If positive for DVT, begin anticoagulation immediately
- You can assume someone has a PE if they have SOB, tachypnea, etc. and have a positive venous Doppler for DVT
- Spiral Chest CTA:
  - Imaging test of choice to diagnose PE if no contraindications such as renal failure or contrast allergy
  - May show RV enlargement and the clot
  - Do if high likelihood based on simplified Wells criteria (see below)
- Lung V/Q scan:
  - For renal failure or contrast allergy
  - If negative, safe to assume no PE if low clinical suspicion as well
- Echo:
  - Not reliable, may show **McConnell's sign** (hypokinesis of RV free wall with normal or hyperkinetic motion of the RV apex) with PE
- Pulmonary angiography:
  - Definitive study, not used much as there is a 0.5% mortality rate
  - Do if catheter-directed thrombolysis is planned

Diagnostic Algorithm:

Simplified Wells criteria for DVT:

- All worth 1 point, except alternative diagnosis at least as likely is -2:
  - Active cancer (Rx ongoing or within 6 months or palliative)
  - Paralysis, paresis, or recent immobilization of lower extremities
  - Recently bedridden for ≥3 days or major surgery within 12 weeks
  - Localized tenderness along distribution of deep venous system
  - Entire leg swelling
  - Calf ≥3 cm larger than other calf (at 10cm below tibial tuberosity)
  - Pitting edema confined to symptomatic leg
  - Collateral superficial veins (nonvaricose)
  - Previous DVT
  - Alternative diagnosis at least as likely as DVT (-2)
- **Score ≤0 → low probability** (5%)
- **Score 1 or 2 → moderate probability** (17%)
- **Score ≥3 → high probability** (53%)

Simplified Wells criteria for PE:

- Alternative diagnosis less likely than PE (3)
- Clinical signs of DVT (leg swelling, pain with palpation) (3)
- Immobilization (bed rest ≥3 days) or surgery within 4 weeks (1.5)
- HR >100 (1.5)
- Prior PE or DVT (1.5)
- Active cancer (1)
- Hemoptysis (1)
- **≤ 4 → unlikely** (13% probability, not high),
- **> 4 → likely** (39% probability, high), **do CT angiogram**

Pulmonary Embolus Rule-out Criteria (PERC):

- Eight criteria, which if the patient fulfills all 8 criteria and has a low probability of a PE, then no further testing. All other patients should get at least a D-dimer.
    - Age <50 years
    - HR < 100
    - Oxyhemoglobin saturation $\geq$ 95%
    - No hemoptysis
    - No estrogen use
    - No prior DVT or PE
    - No unilateral leg swelling
    - No surgery/trauma requiring hospitalization within the prior four weeks

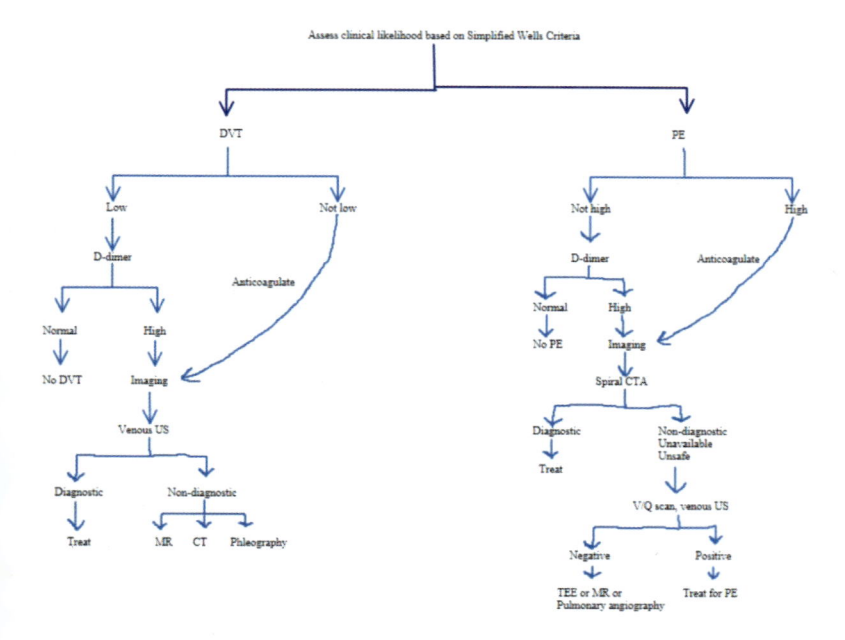

Assess clinical likelihood based on Simplified Wells Criteria

DVT branch:
- Low → D-dimer
    - Normal → No DVT
    - High → Imaging → Venous US
        - Diagnostic → Treat
        - Non-diagnostic → MR, CT, Phlebography
- Not low → Anticoagulate

PE branch:
- Not high → D-dimer
    - Normal → No PE
    - High → Imaging → Spiral CTA
        - Diagnostic → Treat
        - Non-diagnostic / Unavailable / Unsafe → V/Q scan, venous US
            - Negative → TEE or MR or Pulmonary angiography
            - Positive → Treat for PE
- High → Anticoagulate

Pulmonary Embolism Severity Index (PESI) score:

- Once pulmonary embolus has been diagnosed, use this to stratify if the patient is low risk, submassive, or massive to help with what interventions are needed
- Use MDcalc

Treatment:

PE:

- Risk Stratify:
    - Low risk PE → anticoagulation or IVC filter (see below)

- - Submassive → anticoagulation with IR consult for possible IR guided thrombolysis
  - Massive → anticoagulation with IR consult for thrombolysis or embolectomy catheter/surgery
- Supplemental O2 to maintain SaO2 > 92%
- Non-bridge therapy:
  - **NOACs are now preferred for VTE management**
  - Apixaban (Eliquis) 10mg PO BID for 1 week, then 5mg PO BID for 3 months if provoked, at least 6 months if unprovoked, indefinite if 2nd unprovoked
  - Rivaroxaban (xarelto) 20mg PO QD for same duration as above
  - Can't use if kidney dysfunction present
  - **AMPLIFY trial (2013, NEJM)-** Apixaban is noninferior to LMWH and vitamin K antagonist based therapy for VTE recurrence and VTE mortality. Apixaban therapy has a greater reduction in rates of bleeding.
  - **RE-COVER trial (2009, NEJM)-** Among patients with acute VTE, the oral direct thrombin inhibitor dabigatran is as effective as warfarin at reducing recurrence risk, and is associated with less bleeding
  - **AMPLIFY-EXT trial (2013, NEJM)-** In patients with VTE who have completed 6-12 months of anticoagulation, long-term apixaban treatment reduces recurrent VTE or all-cause mortality without increasing rates of major bleeding
  - **EINSTEIN-PE trial (2012, NEJM)-** Among patients with acute PE, rivaroxaban is noninferior to warfarin in preventing recurrent VTE, and is associated with similar bleeding rates
- Bridge therapy:
  - Lovenox (enoxaparin) 1mg/kg subQ Q 12h plus warfarin to get INR 2-3, then discontinue lovenox
  - Unfractionated heparin 80u/kg bolus then 18u/kg/h with warfarin to get INR 2-3 then discontinue heparin
  - Fondaparinux, dosing is weight dependent plus warfarin to get INR 2-3, then discontinue fondaparinux
    - Fondaparinux does not cause heparin induced thrombocytopenia
- IVC filter:
  - Indicated if actively bleeding or recurrent thromboembolism despite adequate anticoagulation or contraindications to anticoagulation
- Fibrinolysis:
  - Only for massive PE that is causing hemodynamic instability and signs of right heart failure
  - tPA 100mg IV over 2h
  - **MOPETT trial (2013, The American Journal of Cardiology)-** For patients with submassive PE, low-dose tPA plus anticoagulation reduced the incidence of pulmonary HTN and of the composite outcome of pulmonary HTN or recurrent PE compared to anticoagulation alone
- Catheter directed fibrinolysis
- Pulmonary embolectomy

DVT:

- Depends on if it is provoked or unprovoked, severity of symptoms, and how many recurrences have occurred
- Distal leg DVTs provoked or unprovoked with mild symptoms do NOT require anticoagulation, and should get follow up ultrasound at 1 and 3 weeks to assess for DVT extension
- Distal leg DVTs provoked or unprovoked with moderate-severe symptoms get anticoagulation (Eliquis 10mg BID for 1 week, then 5mg BID for 3 months)
- Proximal leg DVT provoked or recurrent provoked get 3 months of anticoagulation
- Proximal leg DVT unprovoked gets at least 6 months of anticoagulation
- Proximal leg DVT second time unprovoked gets indefinite anticoagulation
- IVC filter as above
    - **PREPIC trial (1998, NEJM)-** The addition of IVC filter placement to routine anticoagulation for patients with proximal DVT leads to a 4% absolute reduction of PE risk. The modest benefit of IVC filter placement was offset by doubling the rate of recurrent DVT at 2 years.
- Compression stockings replaced every 3-4 months

Etiology:

- Factor V Leiden mutation
- Prothrombin mutation
- Antiphospholipid antibody syndrome
- Cancer
- Obesity
- Smoking
- HTN
- COPD
- CKD
- Long travel
- Oral contraceptives
- Fat embolus
- Tumor embolus
- Bone marrow embolus
- Air embolism
- Amniotic fluid embolus

Risk Factors:

- **Virchows triad:**
    - Stasis- bed rest, CHF, air travel, A-fib
    - Endothelial injury- trauma, surgery, prior DVT, inflammation
    - Thrombophilia- factor V Leiden mutation etc.
- **Prior history of DVT/PE**
- Malignancy
- Age >60
- Obesity
- Pregnancy

- Estrogen use (birth control, HRT)
- Nephrotic syndrome (lose Antithrombin III in urine)

Pathogenesis:

- Virchows triad recruits platelets, which release proinflammatory mediators → platelet aggregation
- Embolization → to lungs or paradoxical embolus to brain (if have PFO)
- Arterial hypoxemia and increased A-a gradient
- Increased dead space → ventilation with no perfusion
- Increased pulmonary vasculature resistance
- Impaired gas exchange → shunting
- Increased airway resistance
- Decreased pulmonary compliance
- Pulmonary HTN → RV wall tension increases → RV dilation and dysfunction (McConnells sign) → increased BNP
- Compression of right coronary artery → ischemia → MI → increased troponins

Complications:

- DVT:
    - PE
    - CVA
    - Postthrombotic syndrome
    - Recurrence
    - Venous stasis/ulcers
    - Phlegmasia alba dolens and cerulen dolens
        - Alba dolens describes a patient with swollen and white leg because of early compromise of arterial flow secondary to extensive DVT
        - Cerulen dolens is considered a precursor of frank venous gangrene. It is characterized by severe swelling and cyanosis and blue discoloration of the extremity.
- PE:
    - Cardiac arrest/death
    - Shock
    - Arrhythmias
    - Pulmonary infarction
    - Pleural effusion
    - Chronic thromboembolic pulmonary HTN
    - Right heart failure
- **Heparin induced thrombocytopenia:**
    - Usually occurs 4-5 days post heparin use
    - Replace heparin with Argatroban as soon as suspected and send HIT panel and serotonin release assay

Admission Orders:

- Admit to floor, ICU if shock/severe cardiopulmonary disease
- Diagnosis DVT or PE
- Condition guarded, critical
- Vital signs Q2h X 4, then Q4h, call for HR >100 or systolic BP <100

- Allergies
- Activity up with assistance, fall precautions
- Nursing O2 by NC to maintain SaO2 >92%, no intramuscular injections
- Diet regular
- Fluids
- Meds:
    - Eliquis 5mg PO BID, or
    - Lovenox 1mg/kg subQ Q 12h with Warfarin per pharmacy
    - Acetaminophen 650mg prn pain
- Labs/diagnostics:
    - CBC
    - CMP
    - Troponins
    - UA
    - PT/INR
    - D-dimer if appropriate
    - EKG
    - CXR
    - CTA, LE Doppler US, echo, if appropriate

Discharge Information:

- Education about anticoagulation
- Nutrition consult before discharge for vitamin K diet if on warfarin
- Follow up on INR if on warfarin
- 30mmHg compression stockings prescription

Additional Notes:

- Important clinical trials:
    - **PESIT trial (2016, NEJM)-** In patients admitted for first episode of syncope, 17% were found to have PE after a standardized, guideline-based inpatient evaluation. PE was identified in 12.7% of patients with an alternative etiology for syncope and 25.4% of patients who did not. PE was identified in 25% of patients without typical signs or symptoms.
    - **AMPLIFY trial (2013, NEJM)-** Apixaban is noninferior to LMWH and vitamin K antagonist based therapy for VTE recurrence and VTE mortality. Apixaban therapy has a greater reduction in rates of bleeding.
    - **RE-COVER trial (2009, NEJM)-** Among patients with acute VTE, the oral direct thrombin inhibitor dabigatran is as effective as warfarin at reducing recurrence risk, and is associated with less bleeding
    - **AMPLIFY-EXT trial (2013, NEJM)-** In patients with VTE who have completed 6-12 months of anticoagulation, long-term apixaban treatment reduces recurrent VTE or all-cause mortality without increasing rates of major bleeding
    - **EINSTEIN-PE trial (2012, NEJM)-** Among patients with acute PE, rivaroxaban is noninferior to warfarin in preventing recurrent VTE, and is associated with similar bleeding rates

- **MOPETT trial (2013, The American Journal of Cardiology)-** For patients with submassive PE, low-dose tPA plus anticoagulation reduced the incidence of pulmonary HTN and of the composite outcome of pulmonary HTN or recurrent PE compared to anticoagulation alone
 - **PREPIC trial (1998, NEJM)-** The addition of IVC filter placement to routine anticoagulation for patients with proximal DVT leads to a 4% absolute reduction of PE risk. The modest benefit of IVC filter placement was offset by doubling the rate of recurrent DVT at 2 years.
- Patients with cancer and thrombosis should be treated with low molecular weight heparin
 - **CLOT trial (2003, NEJM)-** In patients with cancer, dalteparin reduced VTE recurrence without increasing bleeding risk or deaths compared to warfarin

Acute Coronary Syndrome

Definitions:

Acute coronary syndrome encompasses a group of conditions representing myocardial ischemia precipitated by an acute change in myocardial oxygen demand or supply. Stable angina is different in that it is not precipitated by an acute event, but is brought on by predictable exertion, and relieved with short rest in the setting of a stable plaque.

	Unstable Angina	NSTEMI	STEMI	Printzmetal
EKG	ST ↓ T wave inversion Or no EKG changes	ST ↓ T wave inversion Or no EKG changes	ST ↑	ST ↑
Troponins	-	+	+ +	-

History:

When someone is brought in with chest pain, it is important to rule out life threatening situations (aortic dissection, PE, pneumothorax, Mallory Weiss tear, Boerhaave syndrome, etc). The description of the pain is important to help differentiate cardiac pain and non-cardiac pain. It is also important to look for risk factors of ischemic heart disease, such as age, sex, diabetes, HTN, hyperlipidemia, smoking, family history, and obesity. It's also important to note certain populations (diabetics, females) are prone to more atypical presentations (nausea, abdominal pain, etc), and the provider must have a high clinical suspicion in order to treat the condition in a timely manner.

CC:

HPI:

- COLIDDERRS
    - *Typical patient is chest pain worse with exertion, possibly better with rest and nitrates, that is left sided/substernal, non-positional, non-pleuritic, with radiation to the left arm/jaw, non-tender to palpation, in a hypertensive, diabetic, dyslipidemic, smoker, who is old*
- Chest pain description
    - Cardiac pain is usually a pressure or tightness in a retrosternal location
    - Musculoskeletal is usually dull or sharp and reproducible with movement or palpation
    - Pleuritic pain is usually not cardiac in nature
- Location
    - *Can be middle of the chest (retrosternal), upper abdomen, middle back, jaw, left arm*
- Radiation
    - *Typical radiation that may occur is to the left jaw and left arm*
- Duration/severity

- o Unstable angina and NSTEMI usually do not last as long and are not as severe as a STEMI
- o Sense of impending doom can be sign of STEMI
- Pain at rest or with exertion?
  - o *Any acute coronary syndrome can be at rest or with exertion, but if its only with exertion then it is more likely to be unstable angina/stable angina*
- Trauma to the area?
  - o *Usually will be musculoskeletal in nature, or if severe trauma may be myocardial contusion or injury to the aorta*
- Tenderness to palpation?
  - o *Indicative of it being a musculoskeletal injury*
- Positional?
  - o *Indicative of it being a musculoskeletal/pleuritic in nature*
- N/V?
  - o *Can be an atypical presentation of acute coronary syndrome*
- SOB?
  - o *With acute ischemia you can get LV systolic dysfunction leading to pulmonary vascular congestion and SOB*
- Sweating?
  - o *Severe diaphoresis is a sign could be a STEMI*
- Syncope?
  - o *Syncope can be a symptom of acute ischemia*
- History of chest pain?
  - o *What has been done for it in the past?*
  - o *How is this similar?*
  - o *How is this different?*
- Relief with nitroglycerin?
  - o This will relieve pain of unstable angina and NSTEMI, but not STEMI
  - o *This can help you say it is more likely to be acute coronary syndrome, but it can also relieve the pain of diffuse esophageal spasm*
- How far can you walk without stopping? What stops you?
  - o *Baseline activity level and how this is different than that*
- **Diamond Classification:**
  - o This is for the right terminology of the chest pain, whether it is typical, atypical, or non-anginal chest pain. The three characteristics of typical chest pain are:
    - Substernal chest pain
    - Worsened by exertion/stress
    - Relived by nitroglycerin/rest
  - o **Typical** chest pain- has 3/3 of the above
  - o **Atypical** chest pain- has 2/3 of the above
  - o **Non-anginal** chest pain- has <2/3 of the above

ROS:

PMH:

- Hx of Angina?
  - o *And how this may be similar or different than usual, and what has been done for it in the past?*

- Hx of CAD?
    - *And how it was diagnosed, how severe*
- Hx of HTN?
    - *How well controlled it is*
- Hx of Diabetes?
    - *Can present with atypical symptoms for ACS*
- Hx of Hyperlipidemia?
    - *More likely to have plaques in coronaries*
- Hx of CHF?
    - *When was last echo*
- **Hx of recent or current GI bleed?**
    - *Caution with antiplatelet use, have to use clinical judgment*

Surgical H:

- Coronary angiography history? CABG history?

Social H:

- Alcohol, smoking, recreational drugs **(cocaine, meth)**, job, living situation, sexual history
- Menopause?
    - *Women after menopause have a higher risk of mortality from heart disease then men*

Family H:

- Men with MI's at ≤55 years of age
- Women with MI's at ≤65 years of age

Allergies:

Medications:

- Aspirin use?
    - *Important for TIMI risk score*
- Viagra use?
    - *Important because can't give nitrates if taken recently*
- Alpha 2 blocker use?
    - *Important because can't give nitrates if taken recently*

Physical Examination:

A quick thorough exam should be performed, including vitals, in order to rule out life threatening scenarios. If the patient is stable, then signs of cardiac disease should be sought.

- Vitals
    - BP may be hypotensive or hypertensive
        - If suspecting aortic dissection, measure BP in both arms, if there's a difference >20mmHg it may suggest dissection

- Skin
    - Cool sweaty skin can be a sign of myocardial injury
    - Cyanosis can be present in ACS or hypoxia
- Tracheal position
    - Not midline suggests tension pneumothorax
- JVD
    - Can have Kussmaul's sign if there is a RV infarct
        - A rise in jugular venous pressure with inspiration
- Carotids
- Cardiac
    - S3/4, new murmur, tachycardia
    - New or worsening mitral regurgitation may show inferior wall MI
    - New aortic regurgitation may show ascending aortic dissection
- Chest wall palpation
    - Tenderness to palpation highly predicts costochondritis
- Abdominal exam
    - GI reasons are the most common cause of a person coming in with chest pain
- Vascular exam, distal pulses
    - Decreased pulses can show vascular disease and higher risk of heart disease
- Edema
    - Can show RHF, cirrhosis, nephrotic syndrome
- Hepatomegaly
    - Sign of chronic RHF
- Xanthoma
    - Sign of dyslipidemia and shows person has a risk factor for cardiac disease

Differential Diagnosis:

- Stable angina/unstable angina/NSTEMI/STEMI
- Aortic dissection
    - *Sudden onset of severe chest pain, may be anterior chest pain or radiate to the back depending where the dissection is, tearing or ripping pain*
- Pericarditis
    - *More pleuritic chest pain, pain better with leaning forward, pain radiating to trapezius ridge, friction rub murmur, diffuse ST segment elevation and PR segment depression (switched in aVr)*
- Aortic stenosis
    - *Exertional chest pain most likely, crescendo-decrescendo systolic murmur radiating to the carotids*
- PE
    - *More pleuritic chest pain, cough, hemoptysis, hypoxia*
- Cardiomyopathy
    - *Cardiac disease history, enlarged heart, may have EKG changes of LVH or ischemia*
- Myocarditis
    - *Younger person with chest pain, murmur, most likely a recent viral illness*
- Hypertrophic cardiomyopathy

- o *Younger person who gets exertional chest pain, may have syncope with exercise, may have family history of HOCM*
- Pneumonia
    - o *Acute fever/chills, productive cough, pleuritic chest pain, CXR findings*
- Pleuritis
    - o *Lung disease history, smoker, pleuritic pain*
- Pneumothorax
    - o *Pleuritic chest pain, asymmetric breath sounds, CXR findings*
- Bronchitis
    - o *Pleuritic chest pain, hemoptysis, fever, cough*
- GERD
    - o *History of reflux pain (retrosternal pain/burning shortly after eating)*
- Diffuse esophageal spasm **(may be relieved with nitroglycerin just like acute coronary syndrome)**
    - o *Chest pain that may radiate to the jaw, arms, back, dysphagia is common*
- Mallory Weiss tear
    - o *Chest pain, severe vomiting followed by hematemesis, alcoholic*
- Peptic ulcer disease
    - o *Aching or gnawing epigastric pain that can be accompanied by n/v, early satiety, weight loss, maybe NSAID use, alcoholism, or H. pylori history*
- Cocaine use
    - o *Acts to constrict vessels, and can cause acute ischemia with vasoconstriction of the coronary vessels*
- Costochondritis/Tietze syndrome
    - o *Usually trauma associated or exercise, palpation causes pain, position change causes pain*
- Anxiety/panic attack
    - o *SOB, some sort of precipitating event, possible psychiatric history*
- Takatsubo cardiomyopathy
    - o *Usually women, chest pain that is cardiac in nature, can be after emotional event, hypokinesis of the mid and apical left ventricle on ventriculography*
- Thoracic aneurysm
    - o *Pain in the jaw, neck, upper back, coughing, hoarseness, SOB*

Labs:

- CBC
    - o Anemia can cause chest pain, leukocytosis may show infectious process
- CMP
    - o Look for electrolyte abnormalities, LFT's, need to treat hyperglycemia, look for hyperkalemia that needs to be treated
- Troponins x3 Q6h
- BNP
- D-dimer
    - o If low clinical probability from simplified Wells criteria
- CRP

- Lipids
  - Hyperlipidemia/cholesterolemia risk factors for coronary disease
- PT/INR

Imaging:

- EKG
  - ST segment depression in unstable angina and NSTEMI
  - ST segment elevation in STEMI and prinztmetals
  - Look for Q waves, LVH, T wave inversions, tachycardia, heart blocks, etc.
- CXR
  - Can show widened mediastinum in aortic dissection (non-diagnostic)
  - Look for pneumonias, pneumothorax, signs of CHF
- TTE if warranted
  - Looking for pericardial effusion, cardiomegaly, thoracic dissections/aneurysms
- CTA if warranted
  - Based on simplified Wells criteria
  - If suspect aortic dissection/aneurysm

TIMI Risk Score:

- Assesses the risk of cardiovascular events occurring with unstable angina and NSTEMI in the next two weeks. All of the following receive one point **(AMERICA):**
  - $Age \geq 65$
  - **+ M**arkers (cardiac markers troponin, CK-MB)
  - **E**KG changes (ST deviation ≥ 0.5 mm)
  - ≥ 3 **R**isk factors for CAD (see below in risk factors)
  - **I**schemia (≥ 2 angina episodes within 24h)
  - **C**AD history (stenosis $\geq 50\%$)
  - **A**spirin use in past 7 days
- **A score ≥ 3 indicates a benefit of LMWH, GP IIb/IIIa inhibitors, and early angiography**
  - **FRISC-II trial (1999, The Lancet)-** Among intermediate- to high-risk patients with UA/NSTEMI, an early invasive strategy is associated with fewer recurrent MIs and improved long-term survival compared to a non-invasive strategy

Treatment:

Goals of treatment:

- Administer analgesia
  - Morphine, nitroglycerin
- Reduction of myocardial oxygen demand
  - Beta blockers, nitroglycerin, morphine, benzo
- Improvement in coronary blood flow
  - Cath lab, CABG, or thrombolytics
- Prevention of intracoronary thrombosis

- o Aspirin, plavix, enoxaparin, atorvastatin
- **(MONA BASH):**
  - o **M**orphine
  - o **O**xygen
  - o **N**itrates
  - o **A**spirin (best initial treatment for everyone)
  - o **B**eta blocker (not time urgent)
  - o **A**CEI
  - o **S**tatin
  - o **H**eparin
- Order given → O2 → aspirin (325mg) → Nitro → Morphine

Unstable Angina/NSTEMI:

- O2 if SaO2 <90%
- IV access
- Aspirin chewed 325mg, then 81mg PO QD
- Sublingual nitroglycerin 0.4mg 3X in 5 minute intervals (or spray)
  - o Unless have signs of RHF (JVD, edema, crackles), hypotension, HR <50
  - o Also contraindicated if patient has recently taken Viagra or alpha 2 blockers (tamsulosin)
  - o Decreases preload/afterload
- Morphine IV 2-4mg Q5min if pain unresponsive to 3 doses of nitrates
  - o Use cautiously in UA/NSTEMI (some increased mortality)
- Lovenox 1mg/kg SubQ or heparin 60U/kg IV bolus, **urgent**
  - o Lovenox has been shown to be superior to heparin, but it is easy to start a heparin drip as it can be turned off quickly, and monitoring of anticoagulation parameters is measureable
  - o **ESSENCE trial (1997, NEJM)-** Enoxaparin reduces the composite endpoint of death, MI, or recurrent angina at 14 days when compared to UFH in the treatment of UA/NSTEMI
- Beta blockers- IV metoprolol 5mg Q2 min X 3 doses, then 50mg PO Q12h
  - o Contraindicated if HR <50, hypotension, bronchospasm (relative) or signs of RHF (JVD, crackles, edema)
- Atorvastatin 40-80mg QHS (not time urgent)
- Clopidogrel (Plavix) 300mg PO
  - o Unless planning on going to cath lab for PCI, then give ticagrelor (brilinta) 180mg loading dose or prasugrel (effient) 60mg loading dose (has shown to be superior to Plavix), however, most people still use Plavix
  - o **PLATO trial (2009, NEJM)-** Compared to clopidogrel, ticagrelor significantly reduced the rate of CV, MI, or stroke without an increase in the overall rate of major bleeding
  - o **TRITON-TIMI 38 trial (2007, NEJM)-** In patients with ACS and scheduled PCI, prasugrel reduces CV morbidity and mortality but increases bleeding when compared to clopidogrel
- Can give a benzodiazepine to decrease anxiety, thus decreasing heart rate and myocardial oxygen demand
- **Cath lab according to TIMI risk score**
  - o Give a GPIIb/IIIa inhibitor if get stent (abciximab, given in the cath lab)

- Should go to the cath lab within 24 hours, no increased in morbidity or mortality is seen if they are taken to the cath lab within 6 hours compared to 24 hours
- See FRISC-II trial above

STEMI:

- Same as above with these exceptions:
  - **PCI with door to balloon time ASAP (within 90 minutes)**, drug eluting stent
    - Do not allow tests, such as a CXR, to delay reperfusion strategies
  - ACE inhibitor if blood pressure tolerates after reperfusion has been performed
    - **GISSI-3 trial (1994, The Lancet)-** Lisinopril reduces the odds of 6-week mortality by 11% when administered within 24 hours of acute MI
  - Fibrinolysis within 30 minutes of presentation if no PCI is available at the hospital and the closest PCI hospital is ≥ 2 hours away
    - Check fibrinolytic checklist before giving
    - tpA 15 mg bolus then 50mg IV over 30min
    - After thrombolytics given, transfer to PCI center still warranted as reperfusion failure is high with thrombolytics (may need rescue PCI)
    - Give loading dose of plavix (300mg) (prasugrel and ticagrelor have not been studied when thrombolytics have been given)
    - **Contraindications to fibrinolysis**: any prior intracranial hemorrhage, brain tumor/aneurysm/AVM, ischemic stroke within 3 months, active bleeding excluding menses, suspected aortic dissection
  - CABG indications:
    - Significant left main coronary artery stenosis
    - Left main coronary artery equivalent disease- ≥ 70% stenosis of proximal LAD and proximal left circumflex artery
    - Three vessel disease
    - Two vessel disease with significant proximal LAD stenosis and either EF <50% or demonstrable ischemia on noninvasive testing
    - Multivessel disease with diabetes
    - **SYNTAX trial (2009, NEJM)-** CABG resulted in fewer major CV events at 1 year compared with PCI among patients with 3-vessel and/or left main disease
    - **BARI 2D trial (2009, NEJM)-** Among patients with T2DM and stable CAD that are CABG candidates, CABG and OMT reduced the rate of CV events compared to OMT alone. There was no difference in the PCI cohort.
    - **COURAGE trial (2007, NEJM)-** In patients with stable CAD, there were no differences in death and MI between optimal medical therapy plus PCI and OMT alone
    - **EXCEL trial (2016, NEJM)-** Patients with left main CAD and low-intermediate anatomic complexity, PCI

with 2nd generation DES is noninferior to CABG with respect to a primary outcome of death, stroke, or MI at 3 years, though with a nonsignificant trend towards increased mortality
- **FREEDOM trial (2012, NEJM)-** Among diabetic patients with multivessel CAD, revascularization with CABG reduces the rates of death and MI compared to PCI, but causes a modest increase in the rate of stroke
- **STICH trial (2011, NEJM)-** Among patients with ischemic cardiomyopathy with LVEF $\leq 35\%$, the addition of CABG to OMT does not significantly reduce all-cause mortality after 5 years but does reduce CV-related deaths and hospitalizations. After 10 years, there is a significant reduction in all-cause mortality with CABG.
- Post stent medications:
  - Aspirin lifelong
  - Plavix/ticagrelor/prasugrel at least for one year regardless if an intervention was performed. If drug eluting stent, at least one year, and at least one month if bare metal stent (preferred at least one year).
  - **DAPT trial (2014, NEJM)-** Among patients who completed one year of dual antiplatelet therapy (DAPT) after drug-eluting stent PCI, continued DAPT (totaling 30 months) reduces the rate of stent thrombosis and death, MI, or stroke at the cost of increased bleeding

RV/posterior wall infarct:

- See ST elevation in II, III, aVf for inferior (also can include RV), ST depression in V1/V2 for posterior
- Confirm RV infarction with right sided EKG (RV4), look for exam findings
- Elevated JVP, peripheral edema, bradycardia, **classically clear lung fields**
- Do **NOT** give beta blocker, nitroglycerin, or morphine
  - They are preload dependent
- **Give IV fluids** (because they are preload dependent)
- Have atropine ready as the right coronary artery supplies the AV node, so can have symptomatic bradycardia

Printzmetal Angina:

- Calcium channel blockers (especially nifedipine) and nitrates

Etiology:

- CAD
- Atherosclerosis
- HTN
- Embolus (rare)
- Genetics

Risk Factors:

- **Modifiable:**
    - Diabetes
        - Goal A1c <7.0
    - Smoking
    - HTN
        - Goal BP <140/<90
    - Hyperlipidemia
        - Goal LDL <100, better <70
        - Goal HDL >40, better >60
- **Non-modifiable:**
    - Sex (males until after menopause, then females have a higher risk of mortality from heart disease)
    - Family history

Pathogenesis:

- UA/NSTEMI:
    - Imbalance of O2 demand/supply
    - Partially occluding lipid laden thrombus forming on a disrupted atherothrombotic plaque with subsequent intravascular thrombus leading to flow limiting, but non-occlusive subendocardial ischemia leads to ST ↓
    - Coronary spasm, progressive coronary atherosclerosis, increased O2 demand from fever, tachycardia, hypotension, or thyrotoxicosis
- STEMI:
    - Coronary blood flow decreased abruptly after thrombotic occlusion of a coronary artery
    - Plaques prone to rupture have a rich lipid core and a thin fibrous cap
    - Platelet activation → thromboxane A2, fibrin
    - Coagulation cascade activated, factor X activates prothrombin to thrombin, then fibrinogen to fibrin
    - Transluminal fully occlusive ischemia leads to ST ↑
    - Rarely occurs from coronary emboli, congenital abnormalities, or coronary spasm

Complications:

- LV failure
- Cardiogenic shock
    - Decreased CO
    - Hypotension (systolic BP <90)
    - Increased pulmonary capillary wedge pressure (>18 mmHg)
    - Low SCVO2, increased SVR
    - Organ hypoperfusion
- Arrhythmias (most common cause of sudden death after MI)
    - Heart block
    - A-fib
    - Accelerated idioventricular rhythm (benign if within 24 hours)
    - Sinus-brady syndrome
- Mechanical complications

- Free wall rupture
- VSD
- Papillary muscle rupture → mitral regurgitation
- LV thrombus
- Ventricular aneurysms/pseudoaneurysms
    - Persistent ST segment elevation
- Recurrent chest discomfort
- Pericarditis
    - Chest pain relieved by leaning forward, pain radiating to trapezius ridge, friction rub murmur, diffuse ST segment elevation and PR depression
- Dressler syndrome
    - Autoimmune disease with fever, increased ESR, that occurs weeks after the MI

Discharge Information:

- ASA 81mg for life
    - Decreases mortality
- Clopidogrel/prasugrel/ticagrelor regardless if an intervention was performed for at least 1 year
- Beta blocker
    - Decreases mortality
- High dose statin (atorvastatin 40-80mg)
    - **MIRACL trial (2001, JAMA)-** Early initiation of atorvastatin post-UA/NSTEMI reduced the combined endpoint of death, nonfatal MI, cardiac arrest, and ACS requiring hospitalization at 16 weeks, when compared to placebo
    - **PROVE IT-TIMI 22 trial (2004, NEJM)-** After recent ACS, high-dose atorvastatin reduces the rate of CV events compared to moderate-dose pravastatin
    - LDL <100, better <70
    - HDL >40, better >60
- Ezetemibe in addition to statin
    - **IMPROVE-IT trial (2015, NEJM)-** Among individuals with recent ACS, the addition of ezetimibe to moderate-intensity statin therapy is associated with a reduction in CV mortality, major CV event, or nonfatal stroke when compared to statin therapy alone
- Echocardiogram
- ACEI if LVEF <40%
    - Decreases mortality
    - Goal BP <140/<90
- Spironolactone or eplerenone if post-MI and LV EF ≤35% with HF symptoms or diabetes
    - **EPHESUS trial (2003, NEJM)-** Eplerenone reduced the rate of mortality and hospitalizations among patients with acute MI complicated by LV dysfunction and HF symptoms
- Stress test before discharge
- ICD possibly
- Maintain BP <140/90
- Smoking cessation
- Treat diabetes
    - Goal A1c < 7.0

- Exercise 30-60 min 5-7 days/week
- Cardiac rehab
- Weight loss to BMI 18.5-24.9
- Influenza vaccine
- Screen for depression
    - **SADHART trial (2002, JAMA)-** Sertraline is a safe and efficacious treatment for recurrent depression among patients hospitalized for ACS

Admission Orders:

- Admit to cardiac care unit or ICU with telemetry
- Diagnosis STEMI/NSTEMI/UA
- Condition guarded
- Vital signs unit routine, continuous telemetry
- Allergies
- Activity bedrest
- Nursing O2 to maintain SaO2 >92%, IV access, check glucose before each meal and bedtime, call for recurrent chest pain or systolic BP <100 or >180 or HR <50 or >100
- Diet heart healthy
- Fluids depends on fluid status and if signs of RHF or not
- Meds:
    - Aspirin chewed 325mg, then 81mg PO QD
    - Sublingual nitroglycerin 0.4mg 3X in 5 minute intervals
        - Unless have signs of RHF (JVD, edema, crackles), hypotension, HR <50
        - Also contraindicated if patient has recently taken Viagra or alpha 2 blockers (tamsulosin)
    - Beta blockers- IV metoprolol 5mg Q2 min X 3 doses, then 50mg PO Q6h
        - Contraindicated if HR <50, hypotension, bronchospasm (relative) or signs of RHF (JVD, crackles, edema)
    - Morphine IV 2-4mg Q5min
    - Lovenox 1mg/kg SubQ or heparin 60U/kg IV bolus
    - Fluids if have signs of RV or posterior wall MI
    - Atorvastatin 40-80mg QHS, ACEI within 24 hours
    - Clopidogrel (Plavix) 300mg PO
        - Unless planning on going to cath lab for PCI, then give ticagrelor (brilinta) 180mg loading dose or prasugrel 60mg loading dose
    - Cath lab according to TIMI risk score, within 90 minutes on arrival if possible
    - Fibrinolysis within 30 minutes of presentation if no PCI available
        - tpA 15 mg bolus then 50mg IV over 30min
        - Contraindications: any prior intracranial hemorrhage, brain tumor/aneurysm/AVM, ischemic stroke within 3 months, active bleeding except menses, suspected aortic dissection
- Labs/diagnostics:
    - EKG
    - CXR
    - Troponins

- CBC
- CMP
- PT/INR
- Lipids
- Mg/P
- BNP
- D-dimer if indicated

Additional Notes:

- Important clinical trials:
    - **FRISC-II trial (1999, The Lancet)-** Among intermediate- to high-risk patients with UA/NSTEMI, an early invasive strategy is associated with fewer recurrent MIs and improved long-term survival compared to a non-invasive strategy
    - **ESSENCE trial (1997, NEJM)-** Enoxaparin reduces the composite endpoint of death, MI, or recurrent angina at 14 days when compared to UFH in the treatment of UA/NSTEMI
    - **PLATO trial (2009, NEJM)-** Compared to clopidogrel, ticagrelor significantly reduced the rate of CV, MI, or stroke without an increase in the overall rate of major bleeding
    - **TRITON-TIMI 38 trial (2007, NEJM)-** In patients with ACS and scheduled PCI, prasugrel reduces CV morbidity and mortality but increases bleeding when compared to clopidogrel
    - **GISSI-3 trial (1994, The Lancet)-** Lisinopril reduces the odds of 6-week mortality by 11% when administered within 24 hours of acute MI
    - **SYNTAX trial (2009, NEJM)-** CABG resulted in fewer major CV events at 1 year compared with PCI among patients with 3-vessel and/or left main disease
    - **BARI 2D trial (2009, NEJM)-** Among patients with T2DM and stable CAD that are CABG candidates, CABG and OMT reduced the rate of CV events compared to OMT alone. There was no difference in the PCI cohort.
    - **COURAGE trial (2007, NEJM)-** In patients with stable CAD, there were no differences in death and MI between optimal medical therapy plus PCI and OMT alone
    - **EXCEL trial (2016, NEJM)-** Patients with left main CAD and low-intermediate anatomic complexity, PCI with 2nd generation DES is noninferior to CABG with respect to a primary outcome of death, stroke, or MI at 3 years, though with a nonsignificant trend towards increased mortality
    - **FREEDOM trial (2012, NEJM)-** Among diabetic patients with multivessel CAD, revascularization with CABG reduces the rates of death and MI compared to PCI, but causes a modest increase in the rate of stroke
    - **STICH trial (2011, NEJM)-** Among patients with ischemic cardiomyopathy with LVEF $\leq$ 35%, the addition of CABG to OMT does not significantly reduce all-cause mortality after 5 years but does reduce CV-related deaths and hospitalizations. After 10 years, there is a significant reduction in all-cause mortality with CABG.
    - **DAPT trial (2014, NEJM)-** Among patients who completed one year of dual antiplatelet therapy (DAPT) after drug-eluting stent

PCI, continued DAPT (totaling 30 months) reduces the rate of stent thrombosis and death, MI, or stroke at the cost of increased bleeding
- **MIRACL trial (2001, JAMA)-** Early initiation of atorvastatin post-UA/NSTEMI reduced the combined endpoint of death, nonfatal MI, cardiac arrest, and ACS requiring hospitalization at 16 weeks, when compared to placebo
- **PROVE IT-TIMI 22 trial (2004, NEJM)-** After recent ACS, high-dose atorvastatin reduces the rate of CV events compared to moderate-dose pravastatin
- **IMPROVE-IT trial (2015, NEJM)-** Among individuals with recent ACS, the addition of ezetimibe to moderate-intensity statin therapy is associated with a reduction in CV mortality, major CV event, or nonfatal stroke when compared to statin therapy alone
- **EPHESUS trial (2003, NEJM)-** Eplerenone reduced the rate of mortality and hospitalizations among patients with acute MI complicated by LV dysfunction and HF symptoms
- **SADHART trial (2002, JAMA)-** Sertraline is a safe and efficacious treatment for recurrent depression among patients hospitalized for ACS

Heart Failure

Definitions:

Heart failure- inability of the heart to pump sufficient blood to meet the metabolic demands of the body

Heart failure with reduced ejection fraction (HFrEF)- formerly known as systolic heart failure. Primarily occurs from ischemic and non-ischemic cardiomyopathy.

Heart failure with preserved ejection fraction (HFpEF)- formerly known as diastolic heart failure. Primarily occurs from hypertensive, infiltrative, and hypertrophic heart diseases.

Ischemic cardiomyopathy- heart failure caused by ischemia

Non-ischemic cardiomyopathy- heart failure not caused by ischemia

Decompensated heart failure- patients with signs or symptoms of vascular congestion or organ hypoperfusion

Compensated heart failure- patients without signs or symptoms of vascular congestion or organ hypoperfusion

History:

The onset of heart failure is usually gradual, but can be precipitated by certain events (ie. MI). The most common complaints are SOB and fatigue, with peripheral edema occurring with RHF. Symptoms to look for in acute exacerbations are fatigue, SOB, progressive DOE compared to baseline, orthopnea, edema, confusion, and abdominal pain. It is important to find out in the history about 1) functional status 2) weight gain 3) medications 4) recent change in medications 5) last performed echo.

CC:

HPI:

- COLIDDERRS
    - *CHF exacerbation typically shows dyspnea, worsening orthopnea, PND, peripheral edema, crackles, JVD*
- SOB?
    - *Most common symptom of LHF*
- Fatigue?
    - *Common symptom of LHF*
- DOE worse than baseline?
    - *Shows that they may be having an acute exacerbation of their CHF, but could also be COPD exacerbation*
- Orthopnea?
    - Worsening?
    - *Sign of acute exacerbation*
- Nocturnal cough?
    - *Symptom of LHF*

- Paroxysmal nocturnal dyspnea?
    - *Symptom of LHF*
- Sputum production?
    - Pink and frothy
    - *Can be a sign of pulmonary vascular congestion and edema surrounding the bronchi*
- Wheezing?
    - *CHF can cause wheezing to occur from edema around bronchi*
- Confusion?
    - *Sign of inadequate brain perfusion, late sign of CHF*
- Nocturia?
    - *Symptom of RHF*
- Chest pain?
    - *Can be a sign of acute ischemia causing LV failure, which needs to be addressed immediately*
- Edema?
    - *Worsened with prolonged standing, better with leg elevation*
- Early satiety?
    - *Can be a sign of RHF if there is hepatomegaly/ascites*
- Nausea?
    - *Can be a symptom of acute ischemia or RHF from ascites/hepatomegaly*
- Abdominal pain?
    - This is usually overlooked, but if the patient is having abdominal pain, this can be from hepatomegaly or ascites/gut edema from RHF
- History of acute heart failure exacerbations?
    - *What was done for treatment?*
    - *How is this similar?*
    - *How is this different?*

ROS:

PMH:

- Hx of Heart failure?
    - *How was it diagnosed?*
    - *How is it being treated?*
    - *History of exacerbations?*
    - *Last echo?*
- Hx of CAD?
    - *How was it diagnosed?*
    - *How is it being treated?*
- Hx of Diabetes?
    - *How is it being treated?*
    - *Last HbA1c?*
    - *Compliance?*
- Hx of HTN?
    - *How is it being treated?*
    - *Compliance?*
- Hx of Hyperlipidemia?
    - *How is it being treated?*

Surgical H:

Social H:

- Alcohol, smoking, recreational drugs, job, living situation, sexual history

Family H:

Allergies:

Medications:

- If they have a history of heart failure, then **check for medicine compliance**

Physical Examination:

The physical exam will be used to check for fluid status, mental status, pulse pressure, fever, and signs of shock. This will help you determine if the patient is wet or dry, and whether they are warm or cold. This will help you guide your treatment plan in exacerbations.

- Vital signs
    - Hypotension and decreased pulse pressure can be signs of cardiogenic shock
- Labored breathing?
    - Sign of pulmonary vascular congestion
- Sitting vs laying position
    - People with heart failure tend to want to sit up as it helps them breathe
- Cool extremities?
    - This is a feature of cardiogenic shock
- Cyanosis
- JVD (normal is ≤ 8cm)
    - Can be a sign of RHF
- JVD with hepatojugular reflex
    - Putting pressure on the liver increases pressure into the IVC → SVC causing JVD
- Respiratory
    - Crackles, rales, wheezing, Cheynne Stokes respirations
- Cardiac
    - Lateral PMI, S3 (systolic failure, heard with bell), S4 (diastolic failure), murmur, LV heave
- Hepatomegaly
    - Sign of RHF
- Edema
    - Sign of RHF
- Cachexia

Differential Diagnosis:

- Left heart failure:
    - COPD
        - *Causes SOB, DOE, etc. from chronic lung disease just like LHF does*

- o Pneumonia
  - *Causes SOB and DOE, but has an acute onset of fever/chills, productive cough*
- o PE
  - *If large can cause signs of RHF as well as it puts pressure back onto the right heart from the pulmonary vasculature*
  - *SOB is a common symptom*
- Right heart failure:
  - o Cirrhosis
    - *Causes edema, hepatomegaly at first, hypotension, but has other physical exam findings that are more specific to cirrhosis*
  - o Peripheral venous insufficiency
    - *Causes edema and lesions of the bilateral lower extremities, but would not have SOB, hepatomegaly, JVD*
  - o Nephrotic syndrome
    - *Has edema and will have abnormal UA findings*
  - o Myxedema (hypothyroidism)
    - *Will have edema, but will have other features of hypothyroidism (fatigue, obesity, hair thinning, bradycardia, cold intolerance, constipation, decreased reflexes)*
  - o DVT
    - *Will have lower extremity swelling, but usually unilateral*

Labs:

- CBC
  - o Look for anemia → high output HF
  - o May have polycythemia
  - o Look for leukocytosis for possible infectious source of SOB
- CMP
  - o Usually hyponatremic in CHF
  - o Check albumin levels (may be low in CHF or cirrhosis)
  - o Treat hyperglycemia
  - o Correct electrolyte abnormalities
- Troponins
  - o Rule out ischemia as cause of acute CHF exacerbation
- TSH
  - o Look for hypothyroidism causing myxedema
- UA
  - o If have nocturia, polyuria
  - o Also look for microalbumin
- Lipids
  - o Risk factor for coronary disease
- BNP and NT-proBNP
  - o Important to look up prior BNP levels if present
  - o An elevated BNP from baseline is suggestive of an acute exacerbation
  - o Useful to differentiate between dyspnea caused by COPD and CHF
  - o NT-proBNP <300 virtually excludes the diagnosis of HF exacerbation

- Albumin
    - Can help to see if this is due to cirrhosis, may help to see if you need to replace albumin
- ABG if severe respiratory distress
    - Acute flash pulmonary edema may occur and lead to severe respiratory distress, may need to intubate

Imaging:

- EKG
    - Look for arrhythmias or old infarcts
    - Possible acute ischemia causing acute HF exacerbation
- CXR
    - Enlarged heart, cephalization of interstitial markings, Kerley B lines, pulmonary vascular congestion
    - Rule out COPD, pneumonia
- 2D-echo
    - Most useful test
    - **EF**
    - Shows function, anatomy, wall motion, dilation, hypertrophy
    - Can also do a **nuclear** exam, which shows EF and if reversible ischemia is present
    - Pure systolic failure- shows depressed LVEF
    - Pure diastolic failure- shows normal EF, LVH, and abnormal diastolic filling on doppler
- MRI- gold standard for LV mass and volume
- Angiogram if compensated to look for cause
    - Ischemic vs non-ischemic cardiomyopathy
- Right heart cath
    - Confirm elevated pulmonary pressures
    - Not routinely done in in acute exacerbations

New York Heart Association Classification:

Knowing the classification will change the outpatient treatment regimen.

- I- disease with no limitations
- II- disease with slight limitations with physical activity
- III- disease with marked limitation with physical activity
- IV- disease with symptoms at rest

Treatment:

Treatment of Acute Decompensated Heart Failure:

- Supplemental O2 if needed
- Gravity
- Pulmonary edema
    - **Lasix** IV, usually do their home PO dose as the IV dose initially and then titrate from their based on in's/outs
        - **This is the most important intervention**

- o **DOSE trial (2011, NEJM)-** Among patients with acute decompensated HR, high-dose loop diuretics are associated with better symptoms improvement than low-dose loop diuretics at the cost of some renal impairment, while continuous diuretic infusions are no better than intermittent diuretic boluses
  - o Nesiritide infusion for vasodilation
  - o Has **not** been shown to decrease mortality
- Peripheral edema
  - o **Lasix** IV until euvolemic
  - o **This is the most important intervention**
  - o Decreases preload
- Nitropress 3-4mcg/kg/min IV if HTN
  - o Decreased preload
- Morphine 1-3 mg IV Q5 minutes
  - o Decreases preload
- Sit up with legs hanging over bed (decreases preload)
- Hold ACEI if low BP or if Cr >3
- Decrease or hold beta blocker during acute exacerbation
- Cold and wet
  - o Cold is when the patient has altered mental status, fatigue, decreased pulse pressure, or cool extremities
  - o Wet is related to volume status being high
  - o Dobutamine (sys BP >100 and normal diastolic BP), milrinone, dopamine (sys BP 70-100 and bradycardic)
  - o Norepinephrine if sys BP <70
- Cold and dry
  - o Dry is when the patient has warm extremities
  - o Vasodilators (ACEI, CCBs, nitrates)
- Warm and wet
  - o Diuresis as above
- Lovenox 1mg/kg SubQ Q12h
- Fluid/Na restriction
- Intra-aortic balloon pump, ICD, transplant
- Ultrafiltration if needed

Treatment for Chronic HFrEF:

Goal of therapy is to decrease/prevent left ventricular remodeling by controlling excess body water, afterload reduction, and augmentation of contractility (see pathogenesis).

- Neurohormonal antagonism:
  - o ACEI:
    - Benazepril 5-20mg PO QD (or any ACEI)
    - Higher doses as tolerated → decreased hospitalizations (increasing dose does not decrease mortality more)
    - Start this before beta blockers
    - **Decreases mortality**
    - **SOLVD trial (1991, NEJM)-** Enalapril reduces 4-year mortality by 16% and reduces HF hospitalizations when added to conventional therapy in patients with HFrEF
  - o Beta-blockers:

- These are the three proven beta blockers to **decrease mortality**:
  - Carvedilol 6.25-25mg PO BID
  - Metoprolol succinate 12.5-200mg PO QD
  - Bisoprolol 2.5-20mg PO QD
- Can initially worsen symptoms at first, so start them out on low doses then increase (increase slowly, uptitrate every week as tolerated, stop if hypotension or HR <60)
- **COPERNICUS trial (2002, Circulation)-** Carvedilol reduces risk of death or HF hospitalization by 31% compared to placebo in class III-IV HF with EF <25%
- **MERIT-HF trial (1999, The Lancet)-** In patients with symptomatic HFrEF with EF ≤ 40%, long-acting metoprolol led to a 34% reduction in all-cause mortality
- **CIBIS-II trial (1999, The Lancet)-** When added to standard therapy including diuretics and ACE inhibitors, bisoprolol results in a 34% reduction in all-cause mortality in patients with HFrEF (LVEF ≤35%) and NYHA III-IV symptoms
- ARBs:
  - Losartan 25-100mg PO QD, (or any ARB) if can't tolerate ACEIs
  - Don't add if already on an ACEI and beta blocker
  - **Decreases mortality**
  - **Val-HeFT trial (2001, NEJM)-** In a time when HFrEF therapy included ACEI but not beta blockers, addition of valsartan to standard HFrEF therapy did not improve survival but reduced the incidence of the composite endpoint of morbidity and mortality, largely through a decrease in HF hospitalizations
- **The combination of an ACEI/ARB with a beta blocker is better than maxing out one and not being able to start another due to hypotension**
- Mineralcorticoid antagonists:
  - Use for NYHA class II (if EF ≤30%) or III-IV (if EF <35%)
  - Spironolactone 25mg PO QD
    - Decreases mortality
  - Eplerenone 25mg PO QD
  - **EMPHASIS-HF trial (2011, NEJM)-** Eplerenone reduces the risk of death and hospitalization in patients with moderate systolic dysfunction and NYHA class II symptoms
  - **EPHESUS trial (2003, NEJM)-** Eplerenone reduced the rate of mortality and hospitalizations among patients with acute MI complicated by LV dysfunction and HF symptoms
- Arteriovenous dilators:
  - Hydralazine/isosorbide dinitrate 37.5/20 QD
  - Mortality benefit shown in African Americans who were already on ACEI/ARB and beta blocker
  - **A-HeFT trial (2004, NEJM)-** Isosorbide dinitrate plus hydralazine improves survival and reduces hospitalization among African American patients with HFrEF
- Digoxin 3.4-5.1 mcg/kg PO QD
  - Only for symptomatic relief despite optimal hormonal blockade and adequate volume control

- o No decrease in mortality
  - o **DIG trial (1997, NEJM)-** Digoxin reduces hospitalization rate, but does not impact mortality, among patients with HFrEF
- Lasix 20-80mg PO prn
  - o No decrease in mortality, used to control symptoms
- Entresto (sacubitril/valsartan):
  - o Sacubitril inhibits neprilysin which usually increases natrial peptides
  - o Has been **shown to decrease mortality more than an ACEI or ARB alone** in patients with:
    - Stable mild to moderate HFrEF (LVEF $\leq$ 40%)
    - Elevated natriuretic peptide level or hospitalization for HF in the past 12 months
    - Systolic BP $\geq$ 100 mmHg
    - eGFR $\geq$ 20 mL
    - Have tolerated high doses of ACEIs or ARB therapy for $\geq$ 4 weeks
  - o **PARADIGM-HF trial (2014, NEJM)-** Among patients with HFrEF, treatment with an angiotensin receptor-neprilysin inhibitor reduces CV mortality or HF hospitalizations when compared to enalapril. It is also associated with a reduction in all-cause mortality.
- Ivabradine:
  - o Reduces mortality and HF hospitalizations in select patients with NYHA II-IV and LVEF $\leq$ 35% with resting HR $\geq$ 70 BPM despite treatment with evidence based beta blocker (or maximally tolerated beta blocker), ACEI/ARB, and aldosterone antagonists
  - o **SHIFT trial (2010, The Lancet)-** In patients with symptomatic HFrEF (NYHA II-IV) and LVEF $\leq$ 35% with hospitalization for heart failure within the preceding year on contemporary medical therapy (i.e. ACEI/ARB, beta blockers, and aldosterone antagonists) with resting HR $\geq$ 70 BPM, the addition of ivabradine resulted in a 5% absolute reduction in heart failure mortality or hospitalizations at 2 years. The benefit of ivabradine was driven by both a 5% reduction in heart failure hospitalizations as well as a 2% absolute reduction in heart failure mortality.
- Cardiac resynchronization therapy:
  - o For EF $\leq$35% and NYHA class II-IV with QRS $\geq$150ms or LBBB
  - o **MADIT-CRT trial (2009, NEJM)-** Among patients with HF with LVEF $\leq$ 30% and QRS duration $\geq$ 130 msec, placement of an ICD with CRT reduces the rate of mortality or HF events when compared to ICD placement alone. This benefit was driven primarily by a reduction in HF events.
- ICD:
  - o Primary prevention for EF $\leq$35% and NYHA class I-III (NOT IV) for patients who have been on guideline directed medical therapy
  - o **DEFINITE trial (2004, NEJM)-** ICD placement in addition to standard medical therapy was associated with a trend towards decreased mortality among symptomatic patients with moderate non-ischemic dilated cardiomyopathy, LVEF $\leq$ 35%, NSVT, and NYHA class II-III symptoms
- Exercise
- <2g Na a day
- <2L water/day
- Anticoagulation only if needed for other reasons

- **Avoid CCBs, NSAIDs, and TZDs**
- CABG + optimal medical therapy for patients with ischemic cardiomyopathy has shown decreased mortality from all causes over long term (10 years)
    o **STICH trial (2011, NEJM)-** Among patients with ischemic cardiomyopathy with LVEF $\leq$ 35%, the addition of CABG to OMT does not significantly reduce all-cause mortality after 5 years but does reduce CV-related deaths and hospitalizations. After 10 years, there is a significant reduction in all-cause mortality with CABG.

Treatment for Chronic HFpEF:

- Diuretics
- Beta blockers
- BP control
- No nitrates
    o **NEAT-HFpEF trial (2015, NEJM)-** In patients with HFpEF and mild-moderated (NYHA II-III) symptoms, the addition of the long-acting nitrate isosorbide mononitrate appears to hinder rather than improve activity level. Patients on nitrate therapy had a borderline significant reduction in total activity units as well as about a 20-minutes absolute reduction in activity time per day. There was no effect of nitrate therapy on 6-minute walk distance, quality of life, or clinical biomarkers.
- No digoxin
- No therapy has shown a mortality benefit

Treatment of Comorbidities:

- Sleep apnea with CPAP
- Anemia with Fe supplements
- Depression with SSRIs
- Atherosclerosis with high dose statins
- Diabetes with oral meds or insulin

Etiology:

HFrEF ($\leq$40% EF):

- CAD- MI, ischemia
- Pressure overload- mitral regurgitation, aortic regurgitation, aortic stenosis, L$\rightarrow$R shunt
- Chronic lung disease- cor pulmonale, pulmonary vascular disorders
- Non-ischemic dilated cardiomyopathy- familial, infiltrative
- Toxic/drug induced
- Metabolic
- Viral
- Chagas disease
- Arrhythmias- chronic tachy/brady arrhythmias

HFpEF (>40-50% EF):

- Pathologic hypertrophy- primary → hypertrophic cardiomyopathy, secondary → HTN
- Aging
- Restrictive cardiomyopathy- amyloidosis, sarcoidosis, hemochromatosis
- Fibrosis, endomyocardial disorders

High Output States:

- Metabolic- thyrotoxicosis
- Nutritional- Beriberi
- Excessive blood flow requirements- AV shunts, chronic anemia

Risk Factors:

- CAD
- HTN
- Diabetes
- Age
- Men
- Hyperlipidemia
- MI
- Drugs
- Sleep apnea
- Congenital heart defects
- Valvular disease
- Viruses
- Alcohol
- Tobacco
- Obesity
- Arrhythmias

Pathogenesis:

- Progressive, but an index event occurs that damages the heart muscle with loss of myocytes or disruption of the myocardium that decreases generation of force
  - Frank Starling relationship- with exertion in someone with a failing heart, less contractility occurs. So with an increasing preload, the heart cannot produce a large enough stroke volume to accommodate, which produces symptoms
- **Compensatory mechanisms occur**, which may make it asymptomatic for years, but eventually leads to decompensation
  - **Activation of renin-angiotensin-aldosterone system and sympathetic nervous system**, which maintains cardiac output through increased retention of water and salt and vasoconstriction of arterioles to maintain blood pressure (as well as increased endothelin which vasoconstricts vessels)
  - Increased myocardial contractility
  - Increase in vasodilators (ANP, BNP, PGE2, PGI2, NO), that offsets excessive peripheral vasoconstriction

- Transition to symptomatic heart failure is accompanied by increased neurohormonal, adrenergic, and cytokine system activation → **left ventricular remodeling** occurs
    - Myocyte hypertrophy
    - Alterations to contraction properties
    - Progressive loss of myocytes through necrosis, apoptosis, and autophagic cell death
    - Beta-adrenergic desensitization
    - Abnormal myocardial energetics/metabolism
    - Extracellular matrix reorganization to collagen that does not provide structural support to myocytes
- Sustained overexpression of norepinephrine, angiotensin II, TNF alpha, etc, which causes deleterious effects on the heart
- Increased LV mass, volume, and shape occurs from cardiac injury or abnormal hemodynamic loading conditions
- Increased left ventricular end diastolic volume → wall thinning → dilation → decreased stroke volume
    - Hypoperfusion to subendocardium occurs
    - Increased oxidative stress → increase in TNF and IL-1β
    - Sustained expression of stretch activation genes (Ang II, endothelin, TNF) → remodeling
    - Tethering of papillary muscles → mitral regurgitation
- All these mechanical burdens cause left ventricular remodeling, leading to progression of heart failure
- Goal is to prevent/reverse left ventricular remodeling

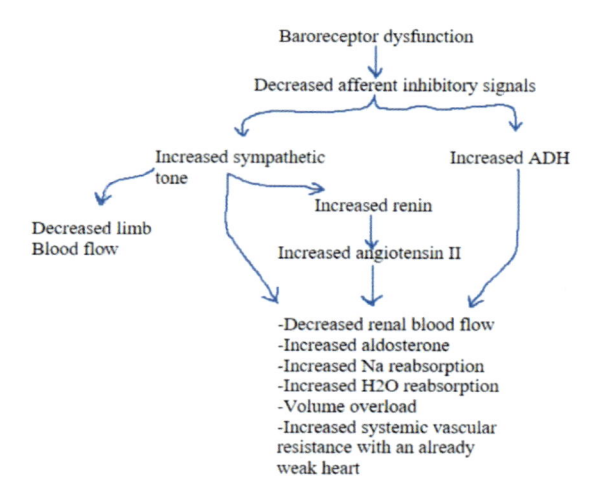

```
Baroreceptor dysfunction
        ↓
Decreased afferent inhibitory signals
    ↙         ↓         ↘
Increased sympathetic           Increased ADH
    tone
  ↙       ↘
Decreased limb    Increased renin
Blood flow            ↓
              Increased angiotensin II
                      ↓
-Decreased renal blood flow
-Increased aldosterone
-Increased Na reabsorption
-Increased H2O reabsorption
-Volume overload
-Increased systemic vascular
 resistance with an already
 weak heart
```

Precipitants of Acute Exacerbation of Heart Failure:

- Dietary indiscretion or medical non-compliance **(40% of causes)**
- Myocardial ischemia/infarction
- Renal failure → increases preload
- Hypertensive crisis
- Worsening aortic stenosis → increases afterload

- Drugs
    - Beta-blockers
    - CCBs
    - NSAIDs
    - TZDs
    - Chemotherapy drugs (**doxorubicin**, trastuzumab)
- Toxins (alcohol, cocaine)
- Arrhythmias
- COPD
- PE
- Mitral regurgitation

Complications:

- Kidney damage or failure (Cardiorenal syndrome)
- Valvular disease
- Arrhythmias
- Cirrhosis
- Death

Admission Orders:

- Admit to telemetry
- Diagnosis acute decompensated heart failure
- Condition guarded
- Vital signs on admit and Q4h, orthostatics Qam, call for RR>30, increasing O2 requirements, systolic BP <95, urinary output <100ml/h
- Allergies
- Activity bedrest with bathroom privileges, up only with assistance, fall precautions
- Nursing daily weights, strict I's/O's, O2 as needed to maintain SaO2 >92%
- Diet 2g Na restriction, heart healthy
- Fluids
- Meds:
    - Lasix IV, initial dose depends on situation
    - Nitropress if hypertensive
    - Hold ACEI/beta-blocker if hypotensive
    - Dobutamine, dopamine, milrinone, or levophed if shock
- Labs/diagnostics:
    - CBC
    - CMP
    - Troponins
    - BNP
    - UA
    - TSH
    - Albumin
    - ABG if severe respiratory distress
    - EKG
    - CXR

Discharge Information:

- Low Na diet
- Importance of medication compliance
- Daily weights with Lasix adjustment prn
- Follow up with PCP and cardiologist
- Prescribe discharge medications that are in treatment of HFrEF section

Additional Notes:

- Important clinical trials:
    - **DOSE trial (2011, NEJM)-** Among patients with acute decompensated HR, high-dose loop diuretics are associated with better symptoms improvement than low-dose loop diuretics at the cost of some renal impairment, while continuous diuretic infusions are no better than intermittent diuretic boluses
    - **SOLVD trial (1991, NEJM)-** Enalapril reduces 4-year mortality by 16% and reduces HF hospitalizations when added to conventional therapy in patients with HFrEF
    - **COPERNICUS trial (2002, Circulation)-** Carvedilol reduces risk of death or HF hospitalization by 31% compared to placebo in class III-IV HF with EF <25%
    - **MERIT-HF trial (1999, The Lancet)-** In patients with symptomatic HFrEF with EF $\leq$ 40%, long-acting metoprolol led to a 34% reduction in all-cause mortality
    - **CIBIS-II trial (1999, The Lancet)-** When added to standard therapy including diuretics and ACE inhibitors, bisoprolol results in a 34% reduction in all-cause mortality in patients with HFrEF (LVEF $\leq$35%) and NYHA III-IV symptoms
    - **Val-HeFT trial (2001, NEJM)-** In a time when HFrEF therapy included ACEI but not beta blockers, addition of valsartan to standard HFrEF therapy did not improve survival but reduced the incidence of the composite endpoint of morbidity and mortality, largely through a decrease in HF hospitalizations
    - **EMPHASIS-HF trial (2011, NEJM)-** Eplerenone reduces the risk of death and hospitalization in patients with moderate systolic dysfunction and NYHA class II symptoms
    - **EPHESUS trial (2003, NEJM)-** Eplerenone reduced the rate of mortality and hospitalizations among patients with acute MI complicated by LV dysfunction and HF symptoms
    - **A-HeFT trial (2004, NEJM)-** Isosorbide dinitrate plus hydralazine improves survival and reduces hospitalization among African American patients with HFrEF
    - **DIG trial (1997, NEJM)-** Digoxin reduces hospitalization rate, but does not impact mortality, among patients with HFrEF
    - **PARADIGM-HF trial (2014, NEJM)-** Among patients with HFrEF, treatment with an angiotensin receptor-neprilysin inhibitor reduces CV mortality or HF hospitalizations when compared to enalapril. It is also associated with a reduction in all-cause mortality.
    - **SHIFT trial (2010)-** In patients with symptomatic HFrEF (NYHA II-IV) and LVEF $\leq$ 35% with hospitalization for heart failure within the preceding year on contemporary medical therapy (i.e. ACEI/ARB, beta blockers, and aldosterone antagonists) with resting

HR $\geq$ 70 BPM, the addition of ivabradine resulted in a 5% absolute reduction in heart failure mortality or hospitalizations at 2 years. The benefit of ivabradine was driven by both a 5% reduction in heart failure hospitalizations as well as a 2% absolute reduction in heart failure mortality.
- **MADIT-CRT trial (2009, NEJM)-** Among patients with HF with LVEF $\leq$ 30% and QRS duration $\geq$ 130 msec, placement of an ICD with CRT reduces the rate of mortality or HF events when compared to ICD placement alone. This benefit was driven primarily by a reduction in HF events.
- **DEFINITE trial (2004, NEJM)-** ICD placement in addition to standard medical therapy was associated with a trend towards decreased mortality among symptomatic patients with moderate nonischemic dilated cardiomyopathy, LVEF $\leq$ 35%, NSVT, and NYHA class II-III symptoms
- **STICH trial (2011, NEJM)-** Among patients with ischemic cardiomyopathy with LVEF $\leq$ 35%, the addition of CABG to OMT does not significantly reduce all-cause mortality after 5 years but does reduce CV-related deaths and hospitalizations. After 10 years, there is a significant reduction in all-cause mortality with CABG.
- **NEAT-HFpEF trial (2015, NEJM)-** In patients with HFpEF and mild-moderated (NYHA II-III) symptoms, the addition of the long-acting nitrate isosorbide mononitrate appears to hinder rather than improve activity level. Patients on nitrate therapy had a borderline significant reduction in total activity units as well as about a 20-minutes absolute reduction in activity time per day. There was no effect of nitrate therapy on 6-minute walk distance, quality of life, or clinical biomarkers.
- Treatment based off of NYHA classes:
    - I- ACEI/ARB + beta blocker
    - II- ACEI/ARB, beta blocker, + Lasix and consider spironolactone
    - III- ACEI/ARB, beta blocker, Lasix, + spironolactone or hydralazine/isosorbide dinitrate
    - IV- same as III, consider transplant with LVAD to bridge, and inotropes, palliative care, **no** ICD
- **Signs/symptoms of left heart failure?**
    - Dyspnea
    - Orthopnea
    - PND
    - Nocturnal cough
    - Confusion and memory impairment
    - Diaphoresis and cool extremities at rest
    - Displaced PMI
    - Increased P2
    - Pulmonary rales (inspiratory crackles)
    - Dullness at the lung bases
    - Left sided S3
    - Left sided S4
    - Left ventricular heave
- **Signs/symptoms of right heart failure?**
    - Elevated jugular venous pressure
    - Ascites/abdominal pain
    - Hepatomegaly/hepatojugular reflex
    - Edema

- Nocturia
    - Right ventricular heave
- A higher level of fruit consumption was associated with lower BP, lower blood glucose levels, with significantly lower risks of major cardiovascular diseases (NEJM Vol 374, NO. 14, pg 1332)

Atrial Fibrillation

Definitions:

<u>Atrial Fibrillation-</u> Disorganized, rapid, and irregular atrial activation with loss of atrial contraction and with an irregular ventricular rate that is determined by AV nodal conduction

<u>Paroxysmal Atrial Fibrillation-</u> episodes that start and stop simultaneously (usually ≤ 48 hours)

<u>Persistent Atrial Fibrillation-</u> longer duration, exceeding 7 days or terminated by treatment

<u>Long-standing persistent Atrial Fibrillation-</u> a-fib that is persistent for more than 1 year

History:

The symptoms of atrial fibrillation (AF) can range from asymptomatic to unstable. If someone has AF that either brings them into the hospital, or occurs while in the hospital or at the office, ask them whether they have had it before. Can they tell if they are in AF when it does happen? Symptoms of AF can be very debilitating on a person's life. It also can lead to strokes, so inquiring about previous or current stroke symptoms is important.

CC:

HPI:

- COLIDDERRS
- Can you tell when you are in AF?
    - *How is this similar?*
    - *How is this different?*
- What symptoms do you get?
    - *How is this similar?*
    - *How is this different?*
- SOB?
    - *Can cause an inadequate ability of the LV to produce an adequate stroke volume, which causes blood to backup into the pulmonary vascular causing congestion*
- DOE?
    - *Same as SOB*
- Angina?
    - *Can cause ischemia due to limited diastolic filling of the coronary arteries*
- Fatigue?
    - *Can be same sensation as SOB and DOE*
- Dizziness?
    - *Arrhythmia causing irregular bloodflow to the brain*
- Syncope?
    - *Arrhythmia causing irregular bloodflow to the brain*
- Palpitations?
    - *Common symptom of AF*

- Slurring of speech?
  - *AF that is not anticoagulated when it should be according to the CHA$_2$DS$_2$-VASC score has a high risk of embolic stroke*
- Weakness?
  - *Stroke symptoms*
- Vision changes?
  - *Embolization to the optical vessels*

ROS:

PMH:

- Hx of Prior stroke?
  - *How is this similar?*
  - *How is this different?*
  - *Medication compliance?*
- Hx of Cardiac disease?
  - *Cardiac disease leads to greater risk of AF*
- Hx of COPD?
  - *Long standing lung disease leads to greater risk of AF*

Surgical H:

Social H:

- Alcohol, smoking, recreational drugs, job, living situation, sexual history

Family H:

Allergies:

Medications:

Physical Examination:

It's important to do a thorough cardiac exam, but also to do a thorough neurological exam.

- Cardiac
  - Irregularly irregular HR
  - Tachycardia
- Neurological
  - Cranial nerves
  - Strength
  - Reflexes, etc.

Differential Diagnosis:

- PAC's
  - *Can feel palpitations, usually benign*
- Atrial flutter
  - *Can feel palpitations, increased risk of stroke, regularly irregular*
- Multifocal atrial tachycardia

- o *Usually long standing lung disease, can have palpitations, tachycardia, at least three P wave morphologies on EKG and HR ≥ 100*
- Sinus tachycardia
    - o *No irregularities on EKG, can have palpitations*
- Sinus arrhythmia
    - o *Different changes in rhythm with inspiration vs expiration, normal variant*
- SVT
    - o *Tachycardia with P waves merging with T waves and difficulty measuring PR interval*
- Wolff Parkinson White syndrome
    - o *Tachycardia with delta waves present*
- V-tach
    - o *Tachycardia with irregular wide QRS*

Labs:

- CBC
- BMP
    - o Check for electrolyte abnormalities that may cause arrhythmias
- Mg
    - o Can cause arrhythmias when deficient, like Torsades de pointes
- Lipids
    - o Risk factor for stroke if have AF
- **TSH**
    - o Hyperthyroidism and hypothyroidism is a common cause of AF

Imaging:

- EKG
    - o **Absent P waves**
    - o **Irregularly irregular rate**
    - o F waves similar to sawtooth pattern in atrial flutter
    - o
- CXR
    - o To exclude COPD, pneumonia, pneumothorax, PE, etc. for SOB
- TTE
    - o Look for LA size, thrombus in LA, valves, EF, and pericardium

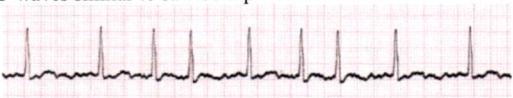

Treatment:

Treatment for New or Recent Onset Atrial Fibrillation:

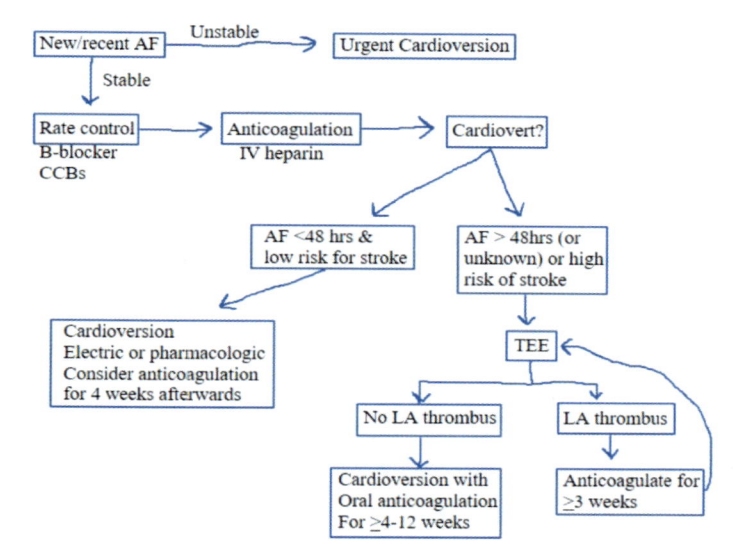

```
New/recent AF --Unstable--> Urgent Cardioversion
       |
     Stable
       ↓
Rate control --> Anticoagulation --> Cardiovert?
B-blocker        IV heparin          /        \
CCBs                                 ↓          ↓
                            AF <48 hrs &    AF > 48hrs (or
                            low risk for    unknown) or high
                            stroke          risk of stroke
                                 ↓               ↓
                            Cardioversion       TEE
                            Electric or         /    \
                            pharmacologic      ↓      ↓
                            Consider       No LA    LA thrombus
                            anticoagulation thrombus   ↓
                            for 4 weeks       ↓      Anticoagulate
                            afterwards    Cardioversion for ≥3 weeks
                                          with Oral
                                          anticoagulation
                                          For ≥4-12 weeks
```

- Heparin or lovenox
- Rate control options:
    - **No CHF Hx → beta blocker or CCB**
    - **CHF Hx → digoxin or amiodarone** (be careful though, amiodarone can convert them and this can result in stroke, should be anticoagulated)
    - Diltiazem IV 0.25mg/kg over 2 minutes, then repeat after 15 minutes 5-15 mg/h infusion
    - Amiodarone IV 150mg bolus over 10 minutes then 0.5-1mg/min x 24h
        - Good if the person is hypotensive or has CHF
    - Metoprolol IV 5mg over 2 minutes, repeat Q5 minutes X 3
    - Verapamil IV 5-10mg over 2 minutes, repeat in 30 minutes
    - Propranolol IV 1mg Q2 minutes
    - Digoxin IV 0.25mg Q2h up to 1.5mg
        - First line if patient has heart failure
- For cardioversion with meds, class III and IC antiarrhythmics can be used
- Cardioversion electrical 200J QRS synchronization shock

Treatment for Chronic/Paroxysmal Atrial Fibrillation:

- **Rate control- goal HR <110 at rest**
    - **Race II trial (2010, NEJM)-** Among patients with permanent AF, lenient rate control (<110 BPM) is as effective as strict rate control (HR <80) in preventing cardiovascular events
    - Metoprolol 25-100mg PO BID or TID

- Propranolol 80-240mg/d divided in doses
- Verapamil 120-360mg/d divided in doses
- Diltiazem 120-360mg/d divided in doses
- Digoxin 0.125-0.375mg QD
- Beta blockers preferred
- If patient has tachycardia induced cardiomyopathy, heart failure, or LVEEF <40%, **can do more stringent rate control (60-80 at rest)**
- Rhythm control
  - No clear survival benefit over rate control
  - **AFFIRM trial (2002, NEJM)-** In patients with nonvalvular AF, there is no survival benefit between rate and rhythm control, but rhythm trends toward increased mortality
- **Anticoagulation-** as the risk for stroke with AF is high
  - Use **CHA$_2$DS$_2$-Vasc** to calculate whether should do anticoagulation
  - Non-valvular AF only:
    - Xarelto (rivaroxaban) 20mg PO QD
    - Eliquis (apixaban) 5mg PO BID
    - Savaysa (edoxaban) 60mg PO QD
    - Pradaxa (dabigatran) 150mg PO BID
  - Warfarin 5mg PO QD with heparin bridge, **goal INR 2-3**
  - **ROCKET AF trial (2011, NEJM)-** Among patients with non-valvular AF, rivaroxaban is noninferior to warfarin in preventing stroke and systemic thromboembolism
  - **ARISTOTLE trial (2011, NEJM)-** In patients with non-valvular AF and at ≥ 1 risk factor, apixaban is associated with a greater reduction in rates of stroke or systemic embolism while having a lower rate of lower bleeding than warfarin
  - **ENGAGE AF-TIMI 48 trial (2013, NEJM)-** Among patients with non-valvular AF, edoxaban is superior to warfarin in preventing stroke or systemic embolism and is associated with lower rates of bleeding and death from CV events
  - **RE-LY trial (2009, NEJM)-** The RE-LY trial demonstrated that compared to warfarin, high-dose dabigatran reduces the stroke risk without increasing the risk of major bleeding among patients with AF, but does increase the risk of GI bleed
  - **AVVEROES trial (2011, NEJM)-** In patients with AF thought to be unsuitable candidates for anticoagulation with a vitamin K antagonist, apixaban significantly reduced the risk of stroke and systemic embolism without increasing the risk of major bleeding or intracranial hemorrhage when compared to aspirin
- Cardioversion
  - Do when hemodynamically unstable, worsening AF, or first ever AF
- Rhythm control if symptomatic despite rate control (improves quality of life)
- Radiofrequency ablation (improves lifestyle, but does not improve survival)
- Surgical maze
- AV node ablation with pacemaker insertion

CHA$_2$DS$_2$-Vasc Score:

Score ≥ 2 → anticoagulate (warfarin, NOACs) (2.2% or higher for stroke)
Score of 1 → consider anticoagulation or just aspirin (1.3% of stroke)
Score of 0 → consider aspirin

- **C**HF (1)
- **H**TN (1)
- **A**ge 65-74 (1)
- **A**ge ≥ 75 (2)
- **D**iabetes (1)
- Prior TIA/**S**troke (2)
- **V**ascular disease (1)
- **S**ex (Female) (1)

HAAS-BLED Score:

Score ≥3 indicates high risk of bleeding, and some caution and regular review of the patient is needed if doing anticoagulation.

- **H**TN history (1)
- **A**bnormal renal function (1)
- **A**bnormal liver function (1)
- **S**troke history (1)
- **B**leeding, prior major bleeding or predisposition to bleeding (1)
- **L**abile INR (1)
- **E**lderly, age > 65 (1)
- m**E**dication usage predisposing to bleeding (antiplatelets, NSAIDs) (1)
- **D**rugs, prior alcohol or drug abuse history (1)

Indications to Admit for New Onset Atrial Fibrillation:

- Patients who ablation of accessory pathway is being considered
- Severe bradycardia after cardioversion
- Treatment for comorbidities that may have caused the new AF (see etiology)
- Elderly patients
- Further manifestations of heart failure or hypotension after control of rhythm or rate

Etiology:

Acute:

- Cardiac:
    - Heart failure
    - Myocarditis or pericarditis
    - Ischemia/MI
    - Hypertensive crisis
    - Cardiac surgery
    - Sick sinus syndrome
    - Pericardial trauma

- Pulmonary:
    - Acute pulmonary disease or hypoxia (COPD flare, pneumonia)
    - PE
    - Sleep apnea
- Metabolic:
    - High catecholamine states (stress, infection, postop, pheochromocytoma)
    - Thyrotoxicosis
    - Hyperthyroidism or hypothyroidism
- Drugs:
    - Alcohol (holiday heart)
    - Cocaine
    - Amphetamines
    - Theophylline
    - Caffeine
- Neurogenic:
    - Subarachnoid hemorrhage
    - Stroke
- Sepsis
- Malignancy

Chronic:

- Increased age
- HTN
- Ischemia
- Valvular disease
- Cardiomyopathies
- Hyper/hypothyroidism
- Obesity

Risk Factors:

- HTN
- Age
- Diabetes
- Cardiac disease
- Sleep apnea
- Male
- Caucasian
- Rheumatic heart disease

Pathogenesis:

- Multiple foci in atria usually near the pulmonary veins fire continuously in a chaotic pattern, causing an irregular rapid ventricular rate
- Atria quiver and do not contract
- Atrial rate ~400, but most are blocked at the AV node → 75-175 BPM
- Blood stasis → clot

Complications:

- **Stroke (causes ~25% of strokes)**
- Heart failure
- Dementia (higher incidence in patients with AF)

Admission Orders:

- Admit to telemetry
- Diagnosis atrial fibrillation
- Condition guarded
- Vital signs Q2h X4, then decreased to Q4h, continuous telemetry
- Allergies
- Activity as tolerated, have patient sit at edge of bed for minutes before standing
- Nursing O2 via NC if SaO2 <93%
- Diet heart healthy
- Fluids
- Meds:
    - Depends on clinical situation, see algorithm above
- Labs/diagnostics:
    - EKG
    - BMP
    - CBC
    - CXR
    - Troponins
    - TSH
    - TTE

Discharge Information:

- If no other diagnosis, discharge when HR controlled
- If discharged on warfarin, education on INR/diet and follow up

Additional Notes:

- Important clinical trials:
    - **Race II trial (2010, NEJM)-** Among patients with permanent AF, lenient rate control (<110 BPM) is as effective as strict rate control (HR <80) in preventing cardiovascular events
    - **AFFIRM trial (2002, NEJM)-** In patients with non-valvular AF, there is no survival benefit between rate and rhythm control, but rhythm trends toward increased mortality
    - **ROCKET AF trial (2011, NEJM)-** Among patients with non-valvular AF, rivaroxaban is noninferior to warfarin in preventing stroke and systemic thromboembolism
    - **ARISTOTLE trial (2011, NEJM)-** In patients with non-valvular AF and at ≥ 1 risk factor, apixaban is associated with a greater reduction in rates of stroke or systemic embolism while having a lower rate of lower bleeding than warfarin
    - **ENGAGE AF-TIMI 48 trial (2013, NEJM)-** Among patients with non-valvular AF, edoxaban is superior to warfarin in preventing

stroke or systemic embolism and is associated with lower rates of bleeding and death from CV events
- **RE-LY trial (2009, NEJM)-** The RE-LY trial demonstrated that compared to warfarin, high-dose dabigatran reduces the stroke risk without increasing the risk of major bleeding among patients with AF
- **AVVEROES trial (2011, NEJM)-** In patients with AF thought to be unsuitable candidates for anticoagulation with a vitamin K antagonist, apixaban significantly reduced the risk of stroke and systemic embolism without increasing the risk of major bleeding or intracranial hemorrhage when compared to aspirin

Syncope

Definitions:

Syncope- Symptom of sudden transient loss of consciousness due to global cerebral hypoperfusion

History:

It is important in cases of pre-syncope or syncope to know about the patients **activity and posture before, during, and after the incident, from BOTH the patient and a witness**. Precipitating factors, prodromes, **postictal states**, and associated symptoms are important. Knowing whether the patient hit their head in cases where the patient fell is important in order to see if cranial imaging is necessary. A history of seizures, as well as narcolepsy and diabetes is important. Lots of medications have been implemented in precipitating syncope as well.

CC:

HPI:

- COLIDDERRS
- Activity and posture before, during, and after incident
- How long were they unconscious?
    - *Longer time unconscious is more likely to be a seizure*
- **What were they like when they woke up?**
    - Confusion after waking up is more likely a seizure
    - Rapid recovery is more likely syncope
- Precipitating factors
    - Exertion- aortic stenosis, hypertrophic cardiomyopathy, pulmonary HTN
    - Positional change- orthostatic
        - *Orthostatic and vasovagal syncope do not occur when they are recumbent, only with sitting or standing*
    - Stressors- sight of blood, pain, emotional distress, fatigue, prolonged standing, warm environment
    - Neurocardiogenic- n/v, cough, micturition, defecation, swallowing
    - Carotid sinus hypersensitivity- head turning or shaving, or wearing a tight tie
    - Subclavian steal- arm activity
- Prodromes
    - Diaphoresis, nausea, blurry vision, warm sensation
    - Cardiac if <5 seconds
    - Vasovagal if >5 seconds
- Associated symptoms
    - Chest pain?
    - Palpitations?
    - Neurologic symptoms?
    - Postictal status (seizures, confusion, etc)
    - Bowel/bladder incontinence?
        - *In syncope, loss of bladder continence is rare, but it is common in seizures*

- Convulsive activity for <10 seconds may mimic seizure activity

ROS:

PMH:

- Hx of prior syncope?
    - *What happened that time?*
    - *How is this similar?*
    - *How is this different?*
- Hx of previous cardiac or neurologic disorders?
    - If no CV disease at baseline, 5% of syncope is cardiac, 25% is vasovagal
    - If CV disease is present, 20% is cardiac, 10% is vasovagal

Surgical H:

Social H:

- Alcohol, smoking, recreational drugs, job, living situation, sexual history

Family H:

- Cardiomyopathies (hypertrophic)?
- Sudden cardiac death (long QT syndrome)?
- Syncope?

Allergies:

Medications:

All of these medications have been implicated to precipitate syncope in some way:

- Diuretics
- Alpha blockers
- Nitrates
- ACEI/ARBs
- CCBs
- Hydralazine
- Phenothiazines
- Antidepressants
- Ganglion blocking agents
- Beta blockers
- Class Ia, IC, or III antiarrhythmics that prolong the QT interval
- Antipsychotics
- Barbituates
- Benzodiazepines

Physical Examination:

Vital signs are important in syncope, as it can diagnose the problem at hand. Other major organ systems to evaluate are cardiac, vascular, and neuro.

- Vital signs
    - Orthostatics, BP, HR, hypoxia (see PESIT trial below for PE)
    - Correct way of doing orthostatics is to let them lay for 5 minutes, then do BP, then then repeat with both sitting and standing
    - Positive if drop in systolic by 20, drop in diastolic by 10, increase in HR by 10-20, or symptoms (unable to stand the entire time)
- Cardiac
    - JVD, PMI, S3, murmurs (AS, MS, MR, HOCM), RV heave with increased P2 (pulmonary HTN)
    - Asses for valvular disorders that can cause syncope
- Vascular
    - Asymmetric pulses, carotid/vertebral subclavian bruits
    - Carotid sinus massage to assess for carotid hypersensitivity (if no bruit)
        - Assess for hypotension (systolic drop by 50) and bradycardia or asystole for 3 seconds
- Neuro
    - Focal findings, tongue bites

Differential Diagnosis:

- Seizure
    - *Long post-ictal confused state, tongue bites, full tonic clonic movements, loss of bowel/bladder function*
- TIA/stroke
    - *Can have unilateral weakness, tingling, slurring of speech, abnormal reflexes*
- Hypoglycemia
    - *Patient takes insulin, found on glucose testing*
- Narcolepsy
    - *History of it, sudden loss of consciousness with stress*
- Vertigo
    - *More dizziness, spinning of the room, no LOC*
- Psychiatric
    - *Psychiatric history, positive drop arm test*

Labs:

- No labs are necessary for all episodes of syncope, it depends on the clinical history
- Glucose for hypoglycemia
    - Easy way to fix/prevent syncope
- CBC
    - Check for anemia
- Troponins, trend
    - Acute ischemia can cause syncope
- BMP

- Check for Na, Ca, K, and Mg which can cause altered mental status or arrhythmias to cause syncope

Imaging:

- EKG/telemetry monitoring for all
  - Look for ischemia, arrhythmias, QT interval, LVH, etc.
- Echo for patients with suspected structural heart disease
  - People with murmurs, family history of sudden cardiac death, syncope during exertion or supine, abnormal EKG (long QRS, AV block type II, sinus pauses, inappropriate bradycardia, nonsustained V-tach, Brugada pattern, Q waves suggesting prior MI, negative T waves in right precordial leads), sudden onset palpitation before syncope
- EEG if indicated
  - If you are suspecting seizures
- CT angiogram or MR angiogram of neck/brain vasculature
  - If you are suspecting neurocardiogenic (vertebrobasilar insufficiency)
- Carotid US if right risk factors (NOT commonly done, however)
  - Can do in hospital, but not commonly done inpatient unless have bruits
- Ambulatory EKG if an arrhythmia is suggested but not recorded (holter, event recorder, loop recorder)
- Exercise treadmill if syncope with exercise
  - Looking for ischemia if CAD suspected
- Tilt table test to exam for vasovagal if it's not cardiac and syncope is recurrent
  - Don't need to do if it's obviously vasovagal in nature
- Electrophysiologic studies if all other studies normal, or if initial workup suggests an arrhythmia, especially if the patient has CAD

Diagnostic Workup:

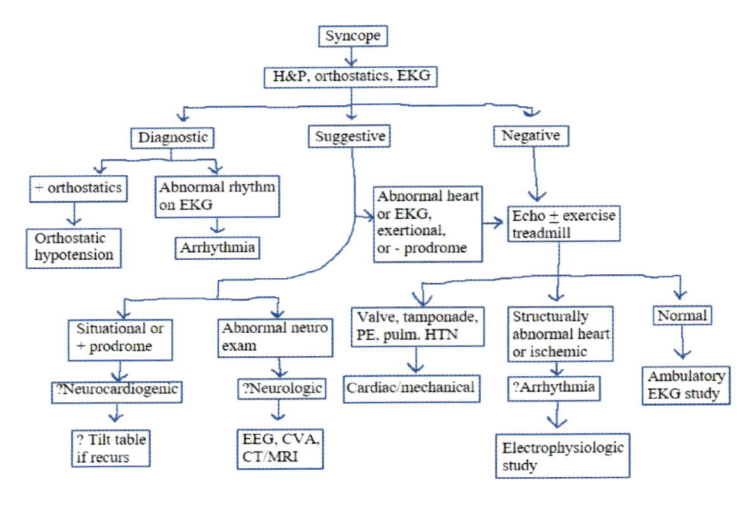

```
                            Syncope
                               ↓
                    H&P, orthostatics, EKG
              ↓            ↓              ↓
         Diagnostic    Suggestive      Negative
         ↓        ↓          ↓             ↓
   + orthostatics  Abnormal rhythm   Abnormal heart
         ↓         on EKG            or EKG,          Echo ± exercise
   Orthostatic       ↓               exertional,     treadmill
   hypotension   Arrhythmia          or - prodrome
                                          ↓               ↓              ↓
                                   Valve, tamponade,  Structurally    Normal
       Situational or  Abnormal neuro  PE, pulm. HTN  abnormal heart
       + prodrome      exam                           or ischemic     ↓
         ↓               ↓                ↓              ↓          Ambulatory
      ?Neurocardiogenic ?Neurologic  Cardiac/mechanical ?Arrhythmia  EKG study
         ↓               ↓                                  ↓
       ? Tilt table   EEG, CVA,                      Electrophysiologic
       if recurs      CT/MRI                         study
```

Historical feature of syncopal episode	Suggested cause(s)
Exertional	Aortic stenosis or mitral stenosis, HOCM, pulmonary HTN
Associated with chest pain	Myocardial ischemia, PE, aortic dissection
Associated with palpitations	Tachy- or bradyarrhythmias
Patient with history of CAD or cardiomyopathy	Ventricular tachyarrhythmia
Family history of syncope or sudden death	Hereditary long QT syndrome, HOCM
Associated with emotional stress, pain, unpleasant auditory or visual stimuli	Vasovagal syncope
Following cough, micturition, or defecation	Situational syncope (form of vasovagal)
After arising from lying or sitting position	Orthostatic hypotension, hypovolemia, autonomic dysfunction
After turning head; during shaving; wearing a tight tie	Carotid sinus sensitivity
Associated with certain body position	Atrial myxoma or 'ball valve' thrombus
Diuretic medication use	Hypovolemia
Antiarrhythmic or anti-psychotic medication use	Ventricular tachyarrhythmias
Parkinson's disease	Autonomic insufficiency
Premonitory aura, tonic-clonic movements, incontinence, long post-ictal state, or tongue biting	Seizure
History of CVA or head trauma	Seizure

VOMAN 321 PE:

- Vasovagal (**vagus nerve overstimulation**):
    - Visceral organs (micturition, defecation, cough, sneeze)
    - Carotid baroreceptors
    - Psychiatric causes (sight of blood, emotional stress)
    - Patient presentation:
        - Situational (pee and pass out a lot, cough or large strain bowel movement and pass out, emotional fight and pass out, wearing a tight tie)
        - Prodrome (dizzy, nauseous, then pass out)
    - Physical exam:
        - Carotid massage with systolic BP decrease of 50 points or asystole for 3 seconds
    - Diagnostic test:
        - Tilt-table test (don't have to do it very often)
- Orthostasis:
    - Volume depleted (diarrhea, dehydration, diuresis, hemorrhage)
    - Dysfunctional autonomic nervous system (diabetes, Parkinsons, elderly, quadriplegic)

- Patient presentation:
  - Orthostatic
- Physical exam:
  - Orthostasis, systolic BP decreased by 20, diastolic BP decreases by 10, HR increased by 10-20, or symptoms (unable to stand to finish exam)
- Diagnostic test:
  - Give IV fluids
    - If it fixes it, it was volume depleted
    - If it doesn't help, they are dysfunctional autonomic nervous system

- **M**echanical cardiac:
  - Valve disorders
  - Patient presentation:
    - Syncope with exertion
    - No prodrome
  - Physical exam:
    - Murmur
  - Diagnostic test:
    - Echo
- **A**rrhythmias:
  - Patient presentation:
    - Sudden in onset
    - No prodrome
  - Physical exam:
    - No physical exam findings
  - Diagnostic exam:
    - EKG with continuous telemetry (observation unit, holter monitor sometimes needed)
    - If it doesn't catch it in observation and still suspicious of arrhythmias as the cause, can do event recorder or loop recorder
- **N**eurogenic (vertebrobasilar insufficiency):
  - Very rare (don't assess for it until you have ruled out every other cause)
  - Patient presentation:
    - Sudden in onset
    - No prodrome
  - Physical exam:
    - Usually no physical exam findings
    - May have focal neurological deficit
  - Diagnostic test:
    - CT angiogram or MR angiogram of blood vessels in back of brain
    - US of carotids usually not best test
- **P**sych (faking it):
  - Patient presentation:
    - Faking it
  - Physical exam:
    - Drop arm test- when they are passed out, lift arm over face and drop, if they move the arm they are faking it, if it hits their face they are not
  - No diagnostic test
- **E**lectrolytes:

- No symptoms
- No physical exam findings
- Diagnostic test:
  - BMP (Na and Ca cause altered mental status, K and Mg lead to arrhythmias)
- Pulmonary Embolism:
  - **PESIT trial (2016, NEJM)**- In patients admitted for first episode of syncope, 17% were found to have PE after a standardized, guideline-based inpatient evaluation. PE was identified in 12.7% of patients with an alternative etiology for syncope and 25.4% of patients who did not. PE was identified in 25% of patients without typical signs or symptoms.

Admittance Criteria:

- **Short version:**
  - Structural heart disease (CHF, MI, CAD)
  - EKG shows an arrhythmia
  - Comorbid reasons (risk factors)
  - Repeat offenders
- Chest pain suggesting ischemia
- Features of CHF
- Moderate-severe valvular disease/cardiac disease
- EKG showing ischemia
- Prolonged QT interval (>500ms)
- Repetitive SA block or sinus pauses
- Persistent sinus brady
- Bi- or trifascicular block or intraventricular conduction delay with QRS >120ms
- Atrial fibrillation
- Non-sustained V-tach
- FmHx of sudden cardiac death
- Pre-excitation syndrome
- Brugada syndrome on EKG (V1-V3 ST concave elevation with T wave inversion, pseudo bundle branch block)
- Palpitations at time of syncope
- Syncope at rest or during exercise

Treatment:

Treatment of Neurally Mediated (vasovagal) Syncope:

- **Reassurance**, avoidance of provocative stimuli and plasma volume expansion with fluid and salt
- Isometric counterpressure maneuvers (leg crossing or handgrip)
- Can go in supine position and elevate legs
- No evidence for fludrocortisone, beta blockers, and vasoconstricting agents

Treatment of Orthostatic Hypotension:

- Remove reversible causes → vasoactive agents
- Increase fluids and salt

- Patient education on moving from supine to upright positions, warnings of large meals, isometric counterpressure maneuvers, raising the head of the bed
- Fludrocortisone acetate 0.1-0.2mg PO QD
- Midodrine 10mg PO TID
- Pseudoephedrine, L-dihydroxyphenylserine, pyridostigmine, yohimbine, DDAVP, erythropoietin

Treatment of Cardiac Syncope:

- Treat the underlying disorder
    - AICD and possibly myomectomy for HOCM
    - Valve replacement for AS and MS
    - Beta blockers, CCBs, or digoxin for SVT
    - Revascularization if ischemia
- Cardiac pacing for sinus node disease and AV block
- Ablation, antiarrhythmics, ICD/defibrillator for atrial and ventricular tachycardias

Etiology:

Neurally Mediated Syncope (most common cause of syncope):

- Vasovagal:
    - Fear, anxiety, emotion, sight of blood, odors
- Situational:
    - Pulmonary- cough, instrument use, weight lifter, sneeze
- Urogenital:
    - Post-micturition, prostatic massage
- GI:
    - Swallowing, CN IX neuralgia, esophageal stimulation, rectal exam, defecation
- Cardiac:
    - Bezold-Jarisch reflex, cardiac outflow obstruction, carotid artery obstruction (unilateral disease is not likely to cause syncope)
- Carotid sinus:
    - Sensitivity, massage
- Ocular:
    - Pressure, exam, surgery

Orthostatic Hypotension:

- Lewy Body disease:
    - Parkinsons, Lewy body, pure autonomic failure
- Multiple system atrophy:
    - Shy Drager syndrome
- Secondary autonomic failure due to autonomic peripheral neuropathies:
    - **Diabetes**, hereditary amyloidosis, primary amyloidosis, hereditary sensory and autonomic neuropathy (HSAN), idiopathic immune-mediated neuropathy, autoimmune autonomic gangliopathy, Sjogrens syndrome, paraneoplastic autonomic neuropathy, HIV, ganglion blocking agents, vasodilators, diuretics
- Postprandial hypotension

- Iatrogenic volume depletion

Cardiac Syncope:

- No aura or prodrome, occurs suddenly (ie patients face hits the floor)
- Arrhythmias:
    - SA node dysfunction, AV node dysfunction, SVT, V-tach, inherited channelopathies
    - Syncope after palpitations suggest arrhythmias
- Cardiac structural disease:
    - Valvular disease (aortic stenosis especially), myocardial ischemia, obstructive and other cardiomyopathies, atrial myxoma, pericardial effusions and tamponade, anomalous coronary artery
- Massive MI
    - Syncope after chest pain suggests acute ischemia
- PE

Cerebrovascular disease:

- Rare cause of syncope
- TIA of vertebrobasilar circulation may lead to syncope

Risk Factors:

- Age
- Female
- Dehydration
- Institutionalized
- Cardiac disease
- Neurologic disease
- Diabetes

Pathogenesis:

- Failure of cerebral blood flow autoregulation mechanisms
- Cessation of blood flow for **~6-8 seconds**
- Decreased CO, decreased peripheral vascular resistance, increased intrathoracic pressure, massive PE, tachy-brady syndrome
- Baroreceptor dysfunction with decreased BP → loss of sympathetic nervous system activation/parasympathetic deactivation, decreased venous return to heart/head

Complications:

- Are secondary to the condition causing it

Admission Orders:

- Admit to telemetry
- Diagnosis syncope
- Condition guarded

- Vital signs telemetry routine, orthostatic BP
- Allergies
- Activity fall risk, up with assistance only
- Nursing O2 to maintain SaO2 >92%, daily weights
- Diet regular
- Fluids Meds:
    - Lovenox
    - Hold lasix
    - Hold meds that can cause syncope (BP meds, diuretics, antidepressants, anti-anginals, analgesics, CNS depressants)
- Labs/diagnostics:
    - CBC
    - BMP
    - Troponins
    - EKG
    - Echo

Discharge Information:

- Holter monitor outpatient if indicated
- Education on sitting to standing and counterpressure maneuvers
- Follow up with PCP

Additional Notes:

- Important clinical trials:
    - **PESIT trial (2016, NEJM)-** In patients admitted for first episode of syncope, 17% were found to have PE after a standardized, guideline-based inpatient evaluation. PE was identified in 12.7% of patients with an alternative etiology for syncope and 25.4% of patients who did not. PE was identified in 25% of patients without typical signs or symptoms.

Upper/Lower GI Bleeding

Definitions:

Upper GI bleed- Intraluminal blood loss from oropharynx to ligament of Treitz

Lower GI bleed- Intraluminal blood loss from ligament of Treitz to anus

History:

A quick history of where and how much blood has been lost is vital to understanding how unstable the patient is. Risk factors for certain conditions that cause bleeding should be assessed, like whether the patient was vomiting prior to an upper GI bleed, if the patient has cirrhosis, any history of varices or prior bleeding episodes, medications that could disrupt the mucosal barrier, etc.

CC:

HPI:

- COLIDDERRS
- Acute or chronic?
    - *Acute has a higher risk of complications and being life threatening*
    - *Chronic is less likely to be life threatening at the moment*
- How much blood has been lost?
    - *Can change the immediate management*
- Prior GI bleeds?
    - *What was done to stop it?*
    - *Was the source found?*
    - *How many times has this happened?*
    - *Is this the same as those other times?*
- Other GI disease?
    - *Can help with knowing if that could be the cause*
    - *How was your GI disease diagnosed and how is it being treated?*
- Hematemesis?
    - *Vomiting blood, suggests upper GI bleed*
    - *Only thing that definitively says it is an upper GI bleed*
- Vomiting prior to hematemesis (Mallory Weiss tear)?
    - *Alcohol use?*
- Coffee ground emesis?
    - *Suggests an upper GI source with slower bleeding rate than hematemesis*
- Melena?
    - *Black, tarry, liquid, foul-smelling stool*
    - *Caused by degradation of hemoglobin by bacteria in the colon*
    - *Presence of melena indicates that blood has remained in the GI tract for several hours*
    - *Dark stools can also result from bismuth, iron spinach, charcoal, and licorice*
    - *90% of the time it is upper GI bleeding*
- Hematochezia?

- o *Bright red blood per rectum, usually represents a lower GI source (typically left colon or rectum)*
  - o *Consider diverticulosis, AVMs, hemorrhoids, and colon cancers*
  - o *It may result from massive upper GI bleeding that is bleeding very briskly*
- Pain?
  - o *Where is it?*
  - o *How severe is it?*
  - o *Radiation?*
  - o *Description of pain?*
- Recent weight loss?
  - o *How much?*
  - o *Unintended?*
  - o *Can be sign of cancer and possibly colon cancer if it's a lower GI bleed*
- Anorexia?
  - o *What happens when you eat?*
  - o *Pain with eating (may be gastric ulcer)?*
- Change in stool caliber?
  - o *What did it used to be like?*
  - o *What is it like now?*
  - o *Tarry?*
  - o *Bright red?*
- Prior abdominal radiation?
  - o *Can cause bleeding as the cells turnover quickly there*

ROS:

PMH:

- Hx of Coagulopathy?
  - o *Can have clots forming in GI vessels and cause acute ischemia with bleeding*
  - o *Can have thin blood easily susceptible to bleeding*
- Hx of Cirrhosis?
  - o *Varices? Prior EGD?*
  - o *Thrombocytopenia, caput medusa then bleeds*
- Risk factors for liver disease?
  - o *Hep B/C? Alpha-1 antitrypsin deficiency? Wilsons disease? Hemochromatosis? Autoimmune hepatitis? Primary biliary cirrhosis?*
- History of cancer?
  - o *Colon cancer particularly*

Surgical H:

- Prior GI or aortic surgeries (post AAA repair)?
  - o *Ischemic colitis common after AAA repair, causes bloody diarrhea and petechial bleeding, insufficient blood supply, especially to watershed areas of colon (splenic flexure)*

Social H:

- Alcohol, smoking, recreational drugs, job, living situation, sexual history

Family H:

Allergies:

Medications:

- Aspirin/NSAIDs?
    - *Risk of peptic ulcers and bleeding as it inhibits formation of prostaglandins which is a mucosal protective barrier*
- Anticoagulants?
    - *Warfarin use, heparin, etc. all predispose to bleeding*
    - *Consider reversal of warfarin with FFP or vitamin K, heparin with protamine*
- Steroids?
    - *Inhibits proper formation of a protective mucosal lining in stomach*

Physical Examination:

Vital signs and the basic ABCs are the most important in cases of upper or lower GI bleed. Peritoneal signs should be sought in case emergent surgery is indicated. Rectal exam is indicated if no obvious frank bleeding is occurring at the present time.

- Vital signs
    - HR and BP, orthostatics
- ABC's
- Nose
    - Look for epistaxis
- Mouth
    - Look for oropharyngeal trauma
- JVP
    - Look at JVP to assess for fluid status
- Abdominal exam
    - Localizable pain, peritoneal signs, hepatosplenomegaly, ascites, caput medusae
- Rectal exam
    - Hemorrhoids, anal fissures, stool appearance, color, occult blood
- Pallor
    - Could suggest anemia and chronicity of bleeding
- Jaundice
    - Can suggest cirrhosis or hemolytic anemias
- Telangiectasias
    - Caput medusa, hemorrhoids
- Spider angiomas
    - Sign of cirrhosis

Differential Diagnosis:

- See etiology

Labs:

- Stool guaiac
    - Positive test only means bleeding is present, does not say if its upper or lower
- CBC (H&H, may be normal at first)
    - Every 4 hours
    - Helps you figure out how brisk the bleeding is
- PT/PTT/INR
    - Helps to determine if they are properly anticoagulated, or too much, and can help to say if they have cirrhosis
- **BUN/Cr ratio**
    - Ratio >36 classically occurs in upper GI bleed because GI resorption of blood (BUN) occurs with ± azotemia
    - In the absence of renal disease, a high BUN suggests GI bleeding
- CMP
    - Look for liver function tests for cirrhosis signs (INR, Cr, albumin, Bili), electrolyte imbalances that may need fixed
- H. pylori testing
    - Common cause of peptic ulcer disease, the most common cause of upper GI bleeds, and a way that antibiotics can help cure the bleeding

Imaging:

- NG tube with lavage (not always done)
    - Fresh blood → active UGIB
    - Coffee grounds → recent UGIB
    - Non-bloody bile → lower source, but does not exclude active UGIB
    - Also helps you quantify how much bleeding there is
- EKG
    - Look for signs of ischemia, arrhythmias
- EGD
    - Performed within 24 hours for UGIB, and possibly for LGIB too
- Anoscopy or proctosigmoidoscopy
- Colonoscopy
    - For LGIB, do EGD 1st occasionally
- Target RBC scan and arteriography, see algorithm to see when to use
    - Definitively located the point of bleeding

Where to Admit:

- ICU:
    - Orthostatics are positive
    - Frankly hypotensive
    - Ongoing obvious hemorrhage
    - Variceal bleed
- Floor:
    - Everyone else with bleed

Diagnostic/Treatment Algorithms:

Tests to order in patients with GI bleed:

- Hematemesis- an upper endoscopy is the initial test
- Hematochezia- first rule out an anorectal cause (ie hemorrhoids). Colonoscopy should be the initial test because colon cancer is the main concern in patients over age 40
- Melena- upper endoscopy is usually the initial test because the most likely bleeding site is in the upper GI tract. Order a colonoscopy if no bleeding site is identified from the endoscopy.
- Occult blood- colonoscopy is the initial test in most cases (colon cancer is the main concern). Order an upper endoscopy if no bleeding site is identified from the colonoscopy.

Approach/Treatment to Upper GI Bleed:

- Endoscopy
- Treatment per GI with IV PPI or drip
- Based on ulcer size and stage (Forrest classification), stay in ICU vs medical floor, vs discharge home, and when to start diet

Approach/Treatment to Lower GI Bleed:

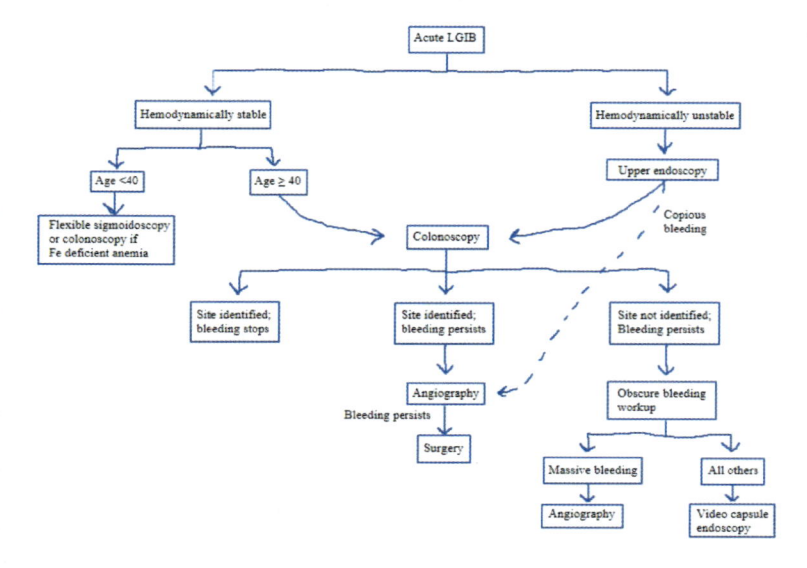

```
                            Acute LGIB
                    ↓                    ↓
        Hemodynamically stable    Hemodynamically unstable
            ↓           ↓                    ↓
        Age <40     Age ≥ 40          Upper endoscopy
            ↓           ↓              ↙  Copious
    Flexible sigmoidoscopy              bleeding
    or colonoscopy if    → Colonoscopy ←
    Fe deficient anemia
                            ↓
            ↓               ↓               ↓
    Site identified;   Site identified;   Site not identified;
    bleeding stops     bleeding persists  Bleeding persists
                            ↓               ↓
                       Angiography ←    Obscure bleeding
                Bleeding persists        workup
                            ↓           ↓         ↓
                        Surgery    Massive      All others
                                   bleeding        ↓
                                      ↓        Video capsule
                                  Angiography  endoscopy
```

Treatment:

Every GI bleed (regardless of location):

- 2 large bore IV's (18 G or larger)

- IV fluid bolus (at least 2L NS)
- Type and cross, transfuse as needed (restrictive transfusion strategy, transfuse Hgb <7)
    - **TRICC trial (1999, NEJM)-** In critically ill patients, restrictive transfusion (Hgb >7) is associated with better survival compared to liberal strategy (Hgb >10)
- IV protonix BID or PPI drip
    - **Omeprazole in Peptic Ulcer Bleeding trial (2000, NEJM)-** This trial demonstrated a 70% reduction in rebleeding with IV omeprazole in patients with active GIB
- GI consult

Treatment of Upper GI Bleed:

- Two large bore IV's (18 G or higher)
- IV NS bolus and type and cross, transfuse Hgb <7)
    - **Transfusion strategies for Acute Upper Gastrointestinal Bleeding trial (2013, NEJM)-** Among patients with acute upper GI bleeding, a restrictive transfusion thereshold (Hgb $\geq$7) was associated with reduced mortality at 45 days compared to a liberal transfusion threshold (Hgb $\geq$10)
        - This trial excluded major GI bleeding, so if patient has major hemodynamically unstable bleed, more liberal transfusion is still warranted
- O2 supplementation
- **Call GI**
- Protonix drip or IV BID
- NG lavage with saline flush
    - If negative, does not mean it is not an upper GI bleed
    - If having a lot of bleeding, makes an EGD more urgent
- If doing endoscopy → erythromycin 250mg IV ~30 minutes before will help with visualization
- Cirrhotic patients:
    - Ceftriaxone IV 1g
    - **Octreotide drip,** 50mcg IV X 1, then 50mcg/h IV X 5 days
        - **This can be lifesaving, so need to inquire about liver disease or variceal disease**
    - **Antibiotics in Cirrhosis with Hemorrhage trial (2006, Gastroenterology)-** Among cirrhotic patients with GI bleed, ceftriaxone reduces the rate of bacterial infection by 67% but does not confer an increased survival benefit when compared to norfloxacin
        - Norfloxacin prevents bacterial infection in cirrhotics with GI hemorrhage (1992)
- **Upper endoscopy**
    - Should be performed within 24 hours in most patients with UGIB
    - Endoscopic therapy, banding, clipping, sclerotherapy, etc.
- NPO
- See etiology for specific treatments

Treatment of Lower GI Bleed:

- Two large bore IV's (18 G or higher)

- IV NS bolus and type and cross
- O2 supplementation
- **Call GI**
- Protonix drip, use if hemodynamically unstable
- If cirrhotic, octreotide drip and ceftriaxone
    - Octreotide drip can be life saving
- NG lavage with saline flush
- If unstable → upper endoscopy or tagged RBC scan
- Colonoscopy after oral lavage solution for most patients
- If massive LGIB → angiography
- Patients <40 years old with minor bleeding → flexible sigmoidoscopy
- Tc labeled red cell scan for 24h may localize bleeding
    - Useful for slow and continuous hemorrhage
- Angiography can detect and treat with embolization (interventional radiology)
    - Do if EGD has copious bleeding, or if EGD is negative but CBC shows brisk bleeding then do this rather than colonoscopy

Etiology/Treatment:

Upper GI Bleed:

- Peptic ulcer disease (~50%, **most common cause):**
    - Burning retrosternal chest pain that then bleeds
    - IV protonix 80 mg IV bolus, then 8mg/h for active, oral if flat or clean base ulcer
    - EGD ± endoscopic therapy
    - Eradicate H. pylori if present
        - Triple therapy including PPI + clarithromycin + (amoxicillin, metronidazole, or levofloxacin)
        - Quadruple therapy (Flagyl + doxycycline + bismuth + PPI)
- Mallory Weiss tears:
    - Self-limiting hematemesis, usually vomiting before in an alcoholic
    - Usually stops spontaneously
    - Endoscopic therapy if active bleeding
- Varices:
    - Hematemesis in a cirrhotic patient
    - If cirrhotic, urgent endoscopy within 12 hours
    - Ceftriaxone IV 1g for 5-7 days
    - **Octreotide drip,** 50mcg bolus and 50mcg/h infusion for 2-5 days
    - Patients with advanced liver disease consider TIPS procedure
    - Propranolol 10-60mg PO TID-QID, start 10mg PO TID, or nadolol
- Hemorrhagic and erosive gastritis:
    - Omeprazole 20mg PO QD X 4-8 weeks
- Boerhaave's:
    - Very sick patient with mediastinitis, SubQ air in the mediastinum (Hammond's crunch), fever, leukocytosis
    - Does NOT present with GI bleed very often, but comparable to Mallory Weiss tears
    - EGD
    - Possible surgery
- Other causes:

- Dieulafoy's lesion (normal anatomic variant that causes an arterial bleed, asymptomatic then painless bleeding)
- Neoplasms
- Osler-Weber-Rendu
- Gastric antral vascular ectasia (GAVE, 'Watermelon stomach')
- Prolapse gastropathy
- Epistaxis
- Oropharyngeal trauma
- Hade's syndrome (upper GI AVM in someone with aortic stenosis)

Lower GI Bleed:

- Diverticular disease **(most common cause):**
    - >50 years old with bad diet with bright red blood per rectum
    - Diverticulosis is painless bleeding
    - Diverticulitis is painful, doesn't bleed as often
    - Spontaneously stops 80% of time
    - Endoscopic treatment (epinephrine, cautery, banding)
    - Arterial vasopressin or embolization
- Angiodysplasia:
    - Usually stops spontaneously
    - Endoscopic therapy
- Hemorrhoids
- Neoplastic (rarely severe bleeding):
    - Weight loss and anemia, FOBT positive
    - A lower GI source of bleeding in a patient over 40 is colon cancer until proven otherwise
- Colitis:
    - Bloody diarrhea, fever, leukocytosis
    - Ulcerative colitis or Crohns disease treatment
- Ischemic colitis:
    - PVD, CAD, CVA, A-fib, post AAA repair, with bloody bowel movements and pain out of proportion to exam
    - Possible colonoscopy or CT scan
    - Resection, surgery
- Postpolypectomy
- Vasculitis

Risk Factors:

- ASA/NSAIDs
- H. pylori
- Alcohol
- Hep B/C
- IV drug abuse
- Low fiber diet
- Steroid use
- Being in the ICU
- Anticoagulants
- Cancer

Complications:

- Death

Admission Orders:

- Admit to
    - ICU for UGIB or LGIB who is unstable or + orthostatics
    - Floor for LGIB unless unstable
- Diagnosis UGIB or LGIB
- Condition
    - Guarded UGIB
    - Stable/guarded LGIB
- Vital signs
    - UGIB- per ICU routine, call for HR >100, systolic BP <100
    - LGIB- Q2h x 2, then Q4h if stable, call for HR > 100, systolic BP <100
- Allergies
- Activity
    - UGIB- bedrest, advanced as tolerated
    - LGIB- ad lib with fall precautions
- Nursing
    - UGIB- place NG tube and lavage to clear, maintain two 18 gauge or larger IV's at all times, strict I's/O's, DVT prophylaxis with SCDs
    - LGIB- place NG tube, aspirate, remove, maintain two 18 gauge IV's, strict I's/O's, DVT prophylaxis with SCDs
- Diet
    - UGIB- NPO initially
    - LGIB- clear liquids then NPO overnight
- Fluids
    - UGIB- NS bolus 2L
    - LGIB- NS bolus prn
- Meds:
    - UGIB:
        - Pantoprazole 80mg IV bolus then 8mg/h for 72h
        - No ASA/NSAIDs
        - If varices or cirrhosis, octreotide 50mcg bolus, then 50mcg/h infusion
        - If cirrhosis, ceftriaxone 1g
        - If cirrhosis, propranolol 10mg PO TID after EGD and stable
        - Erythromycin 250mg IV ~30 minutes before endoscopy
    - LGIB:
        - Go lytely prep
        - No ASA/NSAIDs
- Labs/diagnostics:
    - Same labs for both
    - CBC
    - BUN/Cr
    - PT/PTT/INR
    - CMP
    - EKG
    - H&H Q 2h X 6

o Type and Cross blood

Discharge Information:

- With no evidence or rebleeding for 48-72 hrs

Additional Notes:

- Important clinical trials:
  o **TRICC trial (1999, NEJM)-** In critically ill patients, restrictive transfusion (Hgb >7) is associated with better survival compared to liberal strategy (Hgb >10)
  o **Omeprazole in Peptic Ulcer Bleeding trial (2000, NEJM)-** This trial demonstrated a 70% reduction in rebleeding with IV omeprazole in patients with active GIB
  o **Transfusion strategies for Acute Upper Gastrointestinal Bleeding trial (2013, NEJM)-** Among patients with acute upper GI bleeding, a restrictive transfusion thereshold (Hgb $\geq$ 7) was associated with reduced mortality at 45 days compared to a liberal transfusion threshold (Hgb $\geq$10)
    - This trial excluded major GI bleeding, so if patient has major hemodynamically unstable bleed, more liberal transfusion is still warranted
  o **Antibiotics in Cirrhosis with Hemorrhage trial (2006, Gastroenterology)-** Among cirrhotic patients with GI bleed, ceftriaxone reduces the rate of bacterial infection by 67% but does not confer an increased survival benefit when compared to norfloxacin
    - Norfloxacin prevents bacterial infection in cirrhotics with GI hemorrhage (1992)

Chronic Liver Disease/Cirrhosis Complications

Definitions:

Cirrhosis- histopathologically diagnosed, fibrosis with regenerative nodules

History:

When someone comes to the hospital with chronic liver disease and cirrhosis complications, there are a few things that should come to your attention as to why they are there. 1) **infection**- cirrhotics are more prone to infection 2) **bleeding**- cirrhotics are prone to varices, caput medusa, hemorrhoids, etc. 3) **fluids**- cirrhotics commonly have ascites and peripheral edema, and 4) **medication non-compliance**. All of these need to explored. It is also important to know if the patient has ever had an EGD to look for varices and when their last one was. Also, ask if the patient gets paracentesis', and how often they get them. Mental status is important, as hepatic encephalopathy can be life threatening.

CC:

HPI:

- COLIDDERRS
- Fever/chills?
  - *Spontaneous bacterial peritonitis can be life threatening*
- N/V?
  - *Able to tolerate PO meds or not*
- Abdominal swelling/pain?
  - *Possible SBP and whether you should get a paracentesis, or whether you need to check for peritoneal signs*
- Edema?
  - *Low albumin, possibly CHF*
- Anorexia?
  - *Possibly from ascites pushing up against stomach*
- Change in mental status?
  - *Hepatic encephalopathy*
- Vomit? Blood in vomit?
  - *Varices*
- SOB?
  - *Possible hepatic hydrothorax*
  - *Hepatopulmonary syndrome (platypnea)*
- Dark urine?
  - *Reflux of conjugated bilirubin into the blood is excreted in urine as conjugated bilirubin due to cholestasis being present*
  - *Sign of liver disease, biliary disease, hemolytic anemia, etc.*
- Light stools?
  - *No bilirubin reaches the GI tract (due to reflux into the blood stream from cholestasis), so decreased urobilinogen → decreased stercobilin*
- Itching?
  - *Bile acids deposit in the skin and cause pruritus*

- o *However, levels of bilirubin in the bloodstream and the severity of pruritus does not appear to be highly correlated*
- Fatigue?
    - o *Common symptom of cirrhosis, can be sign of encephalopathy*
- Diarrhea?
    - o *Get diarrhea from cholestasis and cirrhosis*
- Jaundice?
    - o *Buildup of bilirubin in the bloodstream, usually around 2-3 is when jaundice appears (first place is under the tongue)*
- Recent travel?
    - o *Different types of infections can cause cirrhosis, see etiology*
- Recent transfusion?

ROS:

PMH:

- Hx of Cirrhosis?
    - o *When diagnosed?*
    - o *How severe?*
    - o *What is being done for treatment?*
- Hx of Hepatitis B/C?
    - o *Common causes of cirrhosis*
- Hx of CHF?
    - o *Can cause hepatomegaly and liver injury with RHF, and can mimic cirrhosis with symptoms like ascites, peripheral edema, abdominal pain, etc.*
- Hx of Wilsons disease?
    - o *Cause of cirrhosis long term*
- Hx of Hemochromatosis?
    - o *How/when was it diagnosed?*
    - o *How is it being treated?*
- Hx of Alpha-1 antitrypsin deficiency?
    - o *Can cause cirrhosis*

Surgical H:

- Recent surgery?

Social H:

- Alcohol, smoking, recreational drugs (IV drugs), job, living situation, sexual history

Family H:

- Wilsons disease?
- Hemochromatosis?
- Alpha-1 antitrypsin deficiency?

Allergies:

Medications:

- **Compliance** with lasix, beta blocker, lactulose, etc.

Physical Examination:

Knowing the physical exam findings in cirrhosis is important to know. This can either help you make the clinical diagnosis of cirrhosis (even though it's a pathological diagnosis), or help you determine if the patient is decompensating. There are exam findings that are important to look for in every cirrhotic patient, as these findings may point to decompensated disease needing immediate medical attention.

- Vital signs
    - Usually have hypotension, increased pulse pressure
    - Look for fever as can be sign of spontaneous bacterial peritonitis being present
- Blood in mouth
    - Can be sign of bleeding varices
- Respiratory
    - Can have hepatic hydrothorax which can have pleural effusions in the lung bases with dullness to percussion
- Cardiac
    - Cruveilhier-Baumgarten murmur is a venous hum heard in the epigastric region due to collateral connections forming between portal system and the periumbilical veins as a result of portal hypertension
- Abdominal
    - Liver edge (large in early stages, firm/nodular in late stages)
    - Ascites
    - Fluid wave
    - Peritoneal signs
    - Splenomegaly
- Scleral icterus
    - Sign of decompensated cirrhosis
- Palmar erythema
    - Reddening of the palms at the hypothenar and thenar eminences
    - Caused by increase estrogen/nitric oxide
- Parotid gland swelling
    - Usually occurs in cirrhosis caused by alcoholism
    - There is an increase in flow rate, protein, and amylase levels causing hypertrophy of the parotids
- Clubbing
- Edema
    - Low albumin levels
- Decreased body hair
    - From increased estrogen
- Gynecomastia
    - From increased estrogen
- Testicular atrophy
    - From increased estrogen
- Asterixis
    - This is a sign of hepatic encephalopathy

- However, there are 5 stages of hepatic encephalopathy based on severity of symptoms. Asterixis is usually present in stages 2 and 3, and is not present in the most severe stage, 4, where the patient is unconscious. So if this is not present, then it doesn't mean that they do not have hepatic encephalopathy.
- Spider angioma
    - From increased estrogen
- White nails
- Fetor hepaticus
    - Breath smells musty
    - Portal hypertension where portosystemic shunting allows thiols (dimethyl sulfide) to pass directly into the lungs (ketones and ammonia involved too)
- Caput medusa
    - Dilated periumbilical collateral veins due to portal hypertension. Blood from the portal venous system may be shunted through the periumbilical veins and ultimately to the abdominal wall veins (head of Medusa)
- Mental status
    - Assess for hepatic encephalopathy
- Kayser-fleisher rings
    - Copper deposits in the cornea seen in Wilsons disease
- Digital rectal exam to rule out bleeding
- Hemorrhoids
- **Findings that should always be looked for or done:**
    - Oral exam for blood in mouth
    - Abdominal exam for ascites, fluid wave, and peritoneal signs, as this may show that spontaneous bacterial peritonitis is present
    - Asterixis for hepatic encephalopathy
    - Mental status exam for hepatic encephalopathy
    - Presence of caput medusa which is a sign of severe portal hypertension and could be a sign of bleeding
    - Digital rectal exam to rule out bleeding

Differential Diagnosis:

- Edema/ascites:
    - CHF
        - *Peripheral edema, orthopnea, PND, SOB, cardiac history*
    - Nephrotic syndrome
        - *Peripheral edema, no liver disease history, hematuria, abnormal UA*
    - Myxedema
        - *Will have edema, but will have other features of hypothyroidism (fatigue, obesity, hair thinning, bradycardia, cold intolerance, constipation, decreased reflexes, abnormal TSH)*
    - Pancreatitis
        - *Ascites, typical epigastric pain that radiates to the back, alcohol binges, jaundice, n/v, elevated amylase and lipase*
    - Masses

- *Can cause abdominal swelling*
  - (Also see diagnostic workup for SAAG ratio)
- Hepatomegaly:
  - Hepatitis
    - *Can have fever, nausea/vomiting, elevated LFTs*
  - Hepatocellular carcinoma/liver mets
    - *Seen on CT*
  - Right heart failure
    - *Elevated JVP, hepatomegaly, hepatojugular reflex, peripheral edema, nocturia, abdominal pain/ascites*
- Encephalopathy:
  - Uremia
    - *Nausea/anorexia, fibrinous pericarditis, friction rub, asterixis, encephalopathy, bleeding/bruising (platelet dysfunction), increased bleeding time only (not increased PT/INR like in cirrhosis)*
  - Thiamine deficiency
    - *Confusion, ophthalmoplegia, ataxia, confabulation, memory loss (Wernicke Korsakoff syndrome)*
- UGIB:
  - Peptic ulcer disease
    - *Gnawing epigastric pain, possible NSAID use or alcoholism*
  - Mallory Weiss tear
    - *Vomiting before hematemesis, usually alcoholic*
- Non-cirrhotic causes of portal HTN:
  - Portal or splenic vein thrombosis
    - *Seen on CT with contrast*
  - Schistosomiasis
    - *Liver and spleen granulomas and inflammation*

Labs:

- PAN culture (blood culture x 2, UA with culture, sputum culture, CXR)
- CBC
  - Anemia, thrombocytopenia, look for leukocytosis for possible SBP
- CMP
  - Look for electrolyte abnormalities, LFTs, elevated bilirubin
- BUN and Cr
  - Increase in Cr can be sign of acute exacerbation
- PT/PTT/INR
  - Elevated PT and INR is a poor prognostic sign of cirrhosis as all factors except for factor VIII are made in the liver
- Albumin
  - Low albumin usually present as it is made in the liver
- Hepatitis panels
  - Hep A IgM/IgG
    - To see if acute or resolved hep A is/has occurred
  - HBsAg
    - Detectable during acute infection, persistence after 6 months indicates chronic infection
  - HBeAg

- Appears after HBsAg during acute infection, marker of viral replication activity, detectable in chronic infection with high infectivity
    - Anti-HBc IgM
        - Present during acute infection and window phase when both HBsAg and anti-HBs are absent
    - Anti-HBc IgG
        - Detectable along with anti-HBs and anti-Hbe after recovery from acute infection, present without anti-HBs in chronic infection, not present after vaccination (only anti-HBs seen)
    - Anti-HBe
        - Present after recovery from acute infection, HBeAg/anti-HBe seroconversion indicates transition of chronic infection from high to low viral replication and infectivity
    - Anti-HBs
        - Appearance indicates resolution of acute infection, confers long term immunity
    - Hep C RNA
        - To see if hep C is present
- Iron studies
    - Serum Fe, TIBC, TIBC sat %, ferritin
    - Look for hemochromatosis as a possible cause, and if anemia is present to see what type
    - Hemochromatosis has increased serum iron, decreased TIBC, increased ferritin, increased % transferrin saturation (serum iron/TIBC)
- If undiagnosed cause of cirrhosis, get these additional studies:
    - Ceruloplasmin and 24h urinary copper
        - Looking for Wilsons disease
        - Ceruloplasmin will be decreased as it is synthesized in the liver, urinary copper will be increased
    - AMA
        - Checking for primary biliary cirrhosis
    - Anti-smooth muscle
        - Checking for autoimmune hepatitis

Imaging:

- Abdominal US (of kidneys too if increased Cr)
    - Can look for fatty liver, small nodular liver, biliary tree anatomy, presence of ascites
- CXR
    - Looking for pneumonia, cardiomegaly, pleural effusions
- **Paracentesis:**
    - Almost always need to perform on patients who have cirrhosis
    - Especially perform if new onset ascites, worsening ascites, or suspect spontaneous bacterial peritonitis
    - Need to get the **SAAG ratio** (see SAAG ratio workup)
    - Give albumin 6-8 g/L taken off after 5 L are taken off of a large volume paracentesis (e.g., if 3 L taken off, none given, if 6 L taken off, 36-48 g given)

- Possible triple phase abdominal CT scan (look for hepatocellular carcinoma)
- Possible transjugular hepatic biopsy to histologically diagnose cirrhosis

Serum Ascites Albumin Gradient Ratio Workup:

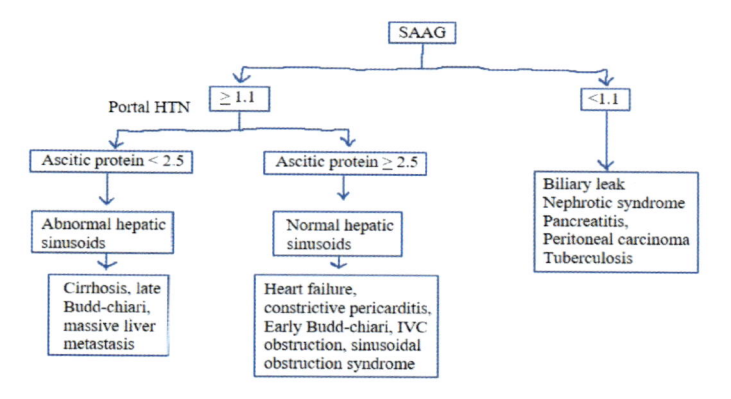

```
                              SAAG
                               |
                ┌──────────────┴──────────────┐
         Portal HTN  ≥ 1.1                  < 1.1
            ┌──────────┴──────────┐           │
   Ascitic protein < 2.5   Ascitic protein ≥ 2.5
            │                     │      Biliary leak
            │                     │      Nephrotic syndrome
   Abnormal hepatic        Normal hepatic   Pancreatitis,
   sinusoids               sinusoids        Peritoneal carcinoma
            │                     │        Tuberculosis
   Cirrhosis, late         Heart failure,
   Budd-chiari,            constrictive pericarditis,
   massive liver           Early Budd-chiari, IVC
   metastasis              obstruction, sinusoidal
                           obstruction syndrome
```

MELD Score:

- Stratifies patients on liver transplant list, and predicts 3 month survival
- Uses Cr, INR, total bili to calculate a score
- >32 → transplant
- **Calculate MELD score every day**

Modified Maddrey's Discriminant Function:

- Stratifies patient with alcoholic hepatitis, and predicts 30 day survival
- Uses PT and Bilirubin
- ≥ 32 → give methylprednisolone

Modified Child-Turcotte-Pugh Scoring System:

Scoring system used to predict 1 year survival and used for transplant evaluation.

	1 point	2 points	3 points
Ascites	None	Easily controlled	Poorly controlled
Encephalopathy	None	Grade 1 or 2	Grade 3 or 4
Bilirubin (mg/dl)	<2	2-3	>3
Albumin (g/dl)	>3.5	2.8-3.5	<2.8
PT (sec>control)	<4	4-6	>6
or INR	<1.7	1.8-2.3	>2.3
Classification			
	A	B	C
Total points	5-6	7-9	10-15
1-yr survival	100%	80%	45%

Complications/Treatment:

- General treatment:
    - Spironolactone 100mg PO QD
    - Lasix 40mg PO QD or IV
    - Multivitamin
    - No narcotics or anxiolytics
    - Lactulose and rifaximin
    - Octreotide and propranolol or nadolol if varices
    - If bleeding, give ceftriaxone
- Portal HTN:
    - Increased hepatic venous pressure to >5mmHg
    - Increased resistance of blood flow through liver, get increased splanchanic blood flow secondary to vasodilation
    - Pre-hepatic- Portal vein thrombosis, splenic vein thrombosis, massive splenomegaly (Bantis syndrome)
    - Hepatic- Schistosomiasis, congenital hepatic fibrosis, cirrhosis, alcoholic hepatitis, veno-occlusive disease
    - Post-hepatic- Budd-chiari, IVC webs, cardiac (restrictive cardiomyopathy, constrictive pericarditis, severe RHF)
- **Variceal hemorrhages:**
    - Blood backs up from portal HTN into gastric veins causing esophageal veins to dilate
    - Screen with endoscopy every 6 months in known cirrhotics
    - Treatment:
        - Endoscopic variceal ligation
        - IV PPI
        - Octreotide drip
        - Prophylaxis with propranolol or nadolol outpatient
        - IV abx (**ceftriaxone, decreases mortality**)
    - **Antibiotics in Cirrhosis with Hemorrhage trial (2006, Gastroenterology)**- Among cirrhotic patients with GI bleed, ceftriaxone reduces the rate of bacterial infection by 67% but does not confer an increased survival benefit when compared to norfloxacin
        - Norfloxacin prevents bacterial infection in cirrhotics with GI hemorrhage (1992)
- **Spontaneous bacterial peritonitis:**
    - Infection of ascitic fluid with 25% in hospital mortality rate
    - E. coli most common cause, if >2 organisms cultured in ascitic fluid, then consider perforated viscus and do exploratory laparotomy
    - Fever, altered mental status, leukocytosis, abdominal pain, but can have no symptoms
    - Paracentesis → **≥ 250 neutrophils/µl**
    - Treatment:
        - Cefotaxime 2g IM/IV Q8h or
        - Ceftriaxone 1g Q12h
        - If not improving, repeat paracentesis at 48 hrs to see if neutrophil count has decreased
        - Albumin after paracentesis (see below), this is also given to prevent hepatorenal syndrome from occurring
        - Albumin Q6h on at least days 1 and 3

- **Effect of Intravenous Albumin on Renal Impairment and Mortality in Patients with Cirrhosis and Spontaneous Bacterial Peritonitis (1999, NEJM)-** In patients with cirrhosis and spontaneous bacterial peritonitis, treatment with intravenous albumin in addition to an antibiotic reduces the incidence of renal impairment and death in comparison with treatment with an antibiotic alone
    - Prophylaxis:
        - Ciprofloxacin or bactrim
- Splenomegaly and hypersplenism:
    - Backup from portal HTN and platelet sequestration
    - Thrombocytopenia, leukopenia, LUQ pain
- Ascites:
    - Accumulation of fluid in the peritoneal cavity
    - Most common cause is from portal HTN
    - Increased abdominal girth, peripheral edema, insidious respiratory compromise → SOB
    - Paracentesis → SAAG ratio
    - Treatment:
        - Decreased Na intake (<2g/day)
        - Free water restriction
        - Spironolactone and furosemide in a 5:2 ratio (eg 100 and 40mg)
            - Goal is to diuresis 1L/day
        - Refractory ascites → large volume paracentesis frequently, TIPS (only used to bridge to a transplant when fatal conditions are present, like varices), transplant
            - Give albumin 6-8 g/L taken off after 5 L are taken off from a large volume paracentesis (e.g., if 3 L taken off, none given, if 6 L taken off, 36-48 g given)
            - **Albumin infusion in patients undergoing large-volume paracentesis: a meta-analysis of randomized trials (2012, Hepatology)-** This meta-analysis provides evidence that albumin reduces morbidity and mortality among patients with tense ascites undergoing large-volume paracentesis, as compared with alternative treatments investigated thus far.
        - Midodrine or clonidine
- Hepatorenal syndrome:
    - Functional renal failure without renal pathology
    - Splanchanic vasodilation occurs in cirrhosis, causing arterial underfilling to occur, which decreases perfusion to the kidneys. This will activate the RAAS system, causing decreased perfusion to the kidneys to occur from vasoconstriction of renal arterioles.
    - Diagnostic criteria:
        - Increase in the serum Cr to >1.5 over days to weeks
        - Lack of response to an albumin challenge of 1 g/kg/d for 2 days
        - Absence of shock, nephrotoxic drugs, active urine sediment, proteinuria >500 mg/d, and US evidence of

parenchymal disease or obstruction, FENa <1%, UNa <10
- Type I- progressive impairment, more severe, doubling of Cr in excess of 2.5 in less than 2 weeks
- Type II- less severe, more gradual increase in Cr
- Treatment:
    - **Best is liver transplant**
    - Midodrine 7.5-125mg PO TID, or levophed if in ICU
    - Octreotide 100-200 mcg SubQ TID
    - IV albumin
    - Terlipressin (rarely used, not available in US)
- **Systematic review of randomized trials on vasoconstrictor drugs for hepatorenal syndrome (2010, Hepatology)-** Terlipressin plus albumin may prolong short-term survival in type 1 HRS. The duration of the response should be considered when making treatment decisions and in the timing of potential liver transplantations. Considering the small number of patients included, the evidence does not allow for treatment recommendations regarding type 2 HRS or any of the remaining treatment comparisons assessed.
- **This does NOT respond to fluid expansion as you would expect**
- DON'T do dialysis, this will just prolong suffering

- Hepatic encephalopathy:
    - Altered mental status and change in cognition in the setting of liver failure
    - Gut derived neurotoxin (ammonium in brain) not removed, goes to brain and causes symptoms
    - Brain edema, cerebral herniation
    - Symptoms range from comatose to violent
    - Occurs from the result of certain precipitants (decreased K+, infection, increased diet in protein, electrolyte imbalances)
    - Grades of hepatic encephalopathy (0-V)
    - Ascites → rule out SBP with paracentesis
    - Asterixis → liver flap, is a classic finding
        - However, this is only found in grades II and III hepatic encephalopathy, and does not occur in 0, I, and IV
        - So can have someone in worst stage of hepatic encephalopathy that does not have asterixis
    - Treatment:
        - Correct electrolytes, fluids, supportive therapy
        - Lactulose 30-45 mL PO TID-QID
            - Colonic acidification causes NH3→ NH4+ conversion, which will be eliminated in feces
            - Goal of therapy is shouldn't be number of bowel movements a day, but is to adjust to correct altered mental status
        - Rifaximin
        - Neomycin, flagyl
        - ± zinc

- Hepatocellular carcinoma:
    - Occurs in 10-25% of cirrhotics
    - Screen with ultrasound Q6 months and AFP

- Hepatic hydrothorax:
    - Pleural effusion caused by ascites usually on right side

- Hepatopulmonary syndrome:
    - **Platypnea** occurs (SOB relieved with lying flat)
    - Vasodilation of pulmonary artery, creates functional right to left shunt
    - 2D echo with bubble study reveals bubbles in 3-6 beats
    - Liver transplant is treatment
- Coagulation disorder:
    - All clotting factors except VIII are made in the liver
    - Treat with FFP and fibrinogen
    - May have same labs as DIC, measure factor VIII, which will be high in liver coagulopathy
- Hyperestrenism:
    - Causes spider angiomas, palmar erythema, gynecomastia, testicular atrophy, hair loss
- Osteoporosis
- Hemorrhoids

Indications for Liver Transplant:

- Primary and secondary biliary cirrhosis
- Primary sclerosing cholangitis
- Autoimmune hepatitis
- Carolis disease
- Cryptogenic cirrhosis
- Chronic hepatitis with cirrhosis
- Hepatic vein thrombosis
- Fulminant hepatitis
    - Acetaminophen, alfa toxin, acute viral hepatitis, autoimmune hepatitis, Budd-chiari, shock liver
- Alcoholic cirrhosis
- Primary hepatocellular malignancies
- Hepatic adenomas
- Non-alcoholic steatohepatitis
- Familial amyloid polyneuropathy

Etiology:

- **Alcohol (60-70%)**- micronodular
- Hep B/C/D chronic (~10%)- IV drug abuse a risk factor
- Autoimmune disease- autoimmune hepatitis
- Metabolic disease- hemochromatosis, wilsons disease, alpha-1-antitrypsin disease
- Biliary tract disease- PBC, secondary biliary cirrhosis (calculus, neoplasm, stricture, atresia), primary sclerosing cholangitis
- Vascular disease- Budd-chiari, right heart failure, constrictive pericarditis, sinusoidal obstruction syndrome
- Non-alcoholic fatty liver disease

Risk Factors:

- See etiology

Pathogenesis:

- Oxidative stress → kuppfer cell activation → cytokines are released and activate stellate cells → increased collagen and fibrosis causing shrinkage of liver

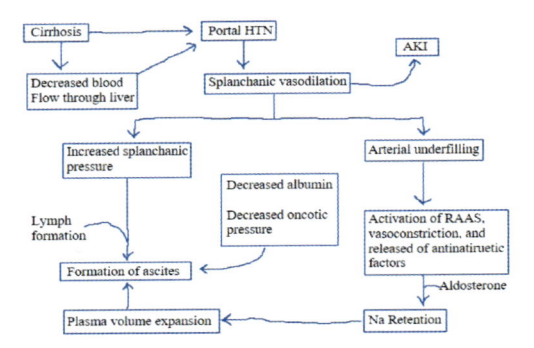

Admission Orders:

- Admit to floor, ICU if gross confusion
- Diagnosis complications of cirrhosis
- Condition fair, adjust accordingly
- Vital signs T, BP, RR, SaO2, neurologic status Q2h X4, then Q4h until stable
- Allergies
- Activity up to commode with assistance and advance as tolerated
- Nursing daily weights, strict I's/O's, SCDs, CIWA protocol if indicated
- Diet low Na
- Fluids none- fluid restriction
- Meds:
    - Spironolactone 100mg PO QD
    - Lasix 40mg PO QD or IV
    - Multivitamin
    - No narcotics or anxiolytics
    - Lactulose and rifaximin
    - Octreotide and propranolol or nadolol if varices
- Labs/diagnostics:
    - CBC
    - CMP
    - UA with culture
    - PA/lat CXR
    - Paracentesis for cell count, differential, and culture

Discharge Information:

- Education on diet/avoidance of toxins/alcohol
- Follow up with GI/hepatology
- Vaccinations for Hep B/C and strep and influenza
- Upper endoscopy screening for varices

- Ultrasound of liver to screen for HCC Q6-12 months

Additional Notes:

- Important clinical trials:
    - **Antibiotics in Cirrhosis with Hemorrhage trial (2006, Gastroenterology)-** Among cirrhotic patients with GI bleed, ceftriaxone reduces the rate of bacterial infection by 67% but does not confer an increased survival benefit when compared to norfloxacin
        - Norfloxacin prevents bacterial infection in cirrhotics with GI hemorrhage (1992)
    - **Effect of Intravenous Albumin on Renal Impairment and Mortality in Patients with Cirrhosis and Spontaneous Bacterial Peritonitis (1999, NEJM)-** In patients with cirrhosis and spontaneous bacterial peritonitis, treatment with intravenous albumin in addition to an antibiotic reduces the incidence of renal impairment and death in comparison with treatment with an antibiotic alone
    - **Albumin infusion in patients undergoing large-volume paracentesis: a meta-analysis of randomized trials (2012, Hepatology)-** This meta-analysis provides evidence that albumin reduces morbidity and mortality among patients with tense ascites undergoing large-volume paracentesis, as compared with alternative treatments investigated thus far
    - **Systematic review of randomized trials on vasoconstrictor drugs for hepatorenal syndrome (2010, Hepatology)-** Terlipressin plus albumin may prolong short-term survival in type 1 HRS. The duration of the response should be considered when making treatment decisions and in the timing of potential liver transplantations. Considering the small number of patients included, the evidence does not allow for treatment recommendations regarding type 2 HRS or any of the remaining treatment comparisons assessed

Acute Pancreatitis

Definitions:

<u>Acute pancreatitis:</u> sudden inflammation of the pancreas which is usually reversible

<u>Chronic pancreatitis:</u> a continuing, chronic, inflammatory process of the pancreas, characterized by irreversible morphologic changes

History:

There are many different causes of acute pancreatitis, all of which should be explored in the history. The severity of the pain also needs to be explored because pain control is a very important factor, but also the extent of inflammation can lead to bacterial infections and necrosis which can be life threatening. A history of pancreatitis can also lead to chronic pancreatitis, which is important in how you treat the disease. A history of recurrent alcoholic pancreatitis is preventable and needs to be addressed.

CC:

HPI:

- COLIDDERRS
    - *Gnawing epigastric pain that radiates to the back, worse with leaning back, relief with leaning forward*
- Abdominal pain severity and location
    - *Usually a severe pain in epigastrium that radiates to the back*
- Radiation of pain?
    - *Usually to the back*
- N/V?
    - *Very common, also need to have IV meds and made NPO*
- Previous attacks?
    - *What was done for it?*
    - *How is this similar?*
    - *How is this different?*
- History of gallstones?
    - *Risk factor for gallstone pancreatitis*
- Alcohol use and if so, recent alcohol binge?
    - *Common risk factor for pancreatitis*
- Hx of hypertriglyceridemia?
    - *Risk factor for pancreatitis*
- Hx of Cystic fibrosis?
    - *Plugs up exocrine glands and can cause pancreatitis*
- Medications (see meds below)
- Recent illness (coxsackie, mumps, EBV, CMV, Hep A, Hep B, TB)?
- ERCP recently?
    - *Pancreatitis occurs in 10-15% of post ERCP patients*
- Trauma?
    - *Can damage the pancreas and cause pancreatitis*
- Scorpion stings?
- Smoker?

- *Smoking a cause of pancreatitis and pancreatic cancer*

ROS:

PMH:

- Hx of previous pancreatitis?
  - *What was done for it?*
  - *How is this similar?*
  - *How is this different?*
- Hx of Gallstones?
  - *Risk factor for gallstone pancreatitis*
  - *What was done for them?*
- Hx of Hypertriglyceridemia?
  - *How high are your values (>1,000)?*
  - *Are you being treated for it?*
- Hx of Cystic fibrosis?
  - *Can cause pancreatitis by plugging up exocrine glands*
- Hx of Cancer?

Surgical H:

- ERCP recently?
  - *Happens in 10-15% of post ERCP patients*

Social H:

- Alcohol, **smoking**, recreational drugs, job, living situation, sexual history

Family H:

Allergies:

Medications:

Lasix, thiazides, sulfonamides, sitagliptin, estrogen, 6-Mercaptopurine, azathioprine, ACEI's, dapsone, 5-ASA, and valproate are all meds that can cause pancreatitis.

Physical Examination:

The amount of distress the person is in can help with severity of the pancreatitis. Hemorrhagic pancreatitis can manifest with specific physical exam findings to help with your diagnosis. It is also important to search for peritoneal signs in case urgent surgery is needed.

- Vital signs
  - Can have a fever, tachycardia, hypotension
- Distress/anxiety
- Jaundice
  - Can be a sign that gallstones may be occurring (choledocholethiasis) or pancreatic head mass
- Scleral icterus

- o   Jaundice from bilirubin accumulation, usually starts at bilirubin 2-3
- Rales
  - o   ARDS is a complication of pancreatitis
- Decreased bowel sounds
  - o   Inflammation of the pancreas can cause bowel peristalsis to decrease
- Abdominal pain and location
  - o   Usually mid epigastric that radiates to the back
- **Cullens sign-** bruising around umbilicus
- **Turners sign-** bruising around flanks
- Hepatomegaly
  - o   Could be sign of pancreatic head mass
- Palpable gallbladder **(Coursovier sign)**
  - o   Sign of pancreatic head mass
- Xanthomas
  - o   Sign of hypertriglyceridemia

Differential Diagnosis:

- Perforated viscus
  - o   *Severe abdominal pain not necessarily in epigastrium, rebound tenderness, free air under the diaphragm on x-ray*
- Acute cholecystitis and biliary colic
  - o   *Pain occurring after meals (especially fatty meals) in the RUQ that can radiate to the R scapula, fever in cholecystitis, see gallstones on US*
- Acute small/large bowel obstruction
  - o   *Abdominal pain with peritoneal signs, rebound tenderness, decreased bowel sounds, KUB shows dilated loops of bowels with fluid levels*
- Mesenteric vascular occlusion
  - o   *Severe abdominal pain that is out of proportion to findings on exam, nausea, bloody stools*
  - o   *If an embolic source, likely has A-fib*
- Renal colic
  - o   *Usually flank pain that radiates to the inguinal area*
- Inferior MI
  - o   *Can present with epigastric pain and nausea, does not radiate to the back, see on EKG with elevated troponins*
- Dissecting aortic aneurysm
  - o   *Older male smoker with hypertension who now has severe abdominal pain and a pulsating palpable mass in the abdomen*
- Pneumonia
  - o   *Can have chest pain that is lower perceived as epigastric pain, would have fever/chills, productive cough*
- DKA
  - o   *Diffuse abdominal pain with n/v/diarrhea and history of diabetes*

Labs:

- CBC

- o May see leukocytosis (part of Ranson criteria, > 16,000), look for anemia (part of Ranson criteria), Hct important (can show hemodilution from severe volume depletion)
- CMP
  - o Look for electrolyte abnormalities and hyperglycemia (part of Ranson criteria, > 200) that needs to be treated and AST levels (AST part of Ranson criteria, >250), BUN/Cr (Ranson criteria)
- Amylase
  - o Levels >450 indicates pancreatic damage
- Lipase
  - o Levels >400 indicates pancreatic damage
- Calcium
  - o Usually hypocalcemia due to saponification, part of Ranson criteria (<8)
- LDH
  - o Part of Ranson criteria, >350
- Bilirubin
  - o Trying to see if liver/biliary function is abnormal
- CRP
  - o Looks for inflammation, good to trend this
- Lipids
  - o Triglycerides >1000 a risk factor
- PT/PTT/INR
  - o Look for liver function and if they are susceptible to bleeding

Imaging:

- Abdominal US- **initial test**, to see gallstones/bile duct dilation, pseudocysts
- Abdominal CT- **test of choice**, not necessary however to diagnose pancreatitis, can consider if not improving after 48-72 hours
- KUB/CXR- sentinel loop, air in small bowel in LUQ, atelectasis, pleural effusion
- Endoscopic ultrasound/MRCP- replacing ERCP for diagnostics

Diagnostic Criteria:

Need **two of the following three** to diagnose acute pancreatitis:

- Typical abdominal pain in epigastrium radiating to the back
- 3X or greater elevation in serum lipase and/or amylase
- Confirmatory findings of acute pancreatitis on CT
  - o Focal or diffuse parenchymal enlargement
  - o Changes in density because of edema
  - o Indistinct pancreatic margins owing to inflammation
  - o Surrounding retroperitoneal fat stranding
  - o Liquefactive necrosis (lack of parenchymal enhancement)
  - o Infected necrosis
  - o Abscess formation
  - o Hemorrhage

Prognostic Criteria:

APACHE II:

Severe if score ≥ 8 (use MD calc). This is the **BEST scoring system for prognosis.** You can use this on both admission and on a daily basis to assess the patients prognosis and response to treatment.

Ranson's Criteria:

Ranson's criteria for pancreatitis estimates mortality of patients with pancreatitis based on initial and 48 hour lab values.

- At diagnosis:
    - Age ≥ 55
    - WBC ≥ 16,000
    - Glucose ≥ 200
    - AST ≥ 250
    - LDH ≥ 350
- At 48 hours:
    - Hct decreased ≥ 10%
    - BUN increased ≥ 5
    - Base deficit > 4
    - Ca < 8
    - PaO2 < 60
    - Fluid sequestration > 6L
- Prognosis and mortality:
    - ≤ 2 → <5%
    - 3-4 → 15-20%
    - 5-6 → 40%
    - ≥ 7 → >99%

BISAP:

- 5 point scoring system on admission:
    - BUN > 25
    - GCS < 15
    - SIRS
    - Age > 60
    - Pleural effusion
- Higher points, higher mortality
- ≥ 3 → ICU admission

CT severity index:

Use MD calc

Treatment:

85-90% are self-limited and subside spontaneously

- Aggressive fluids:

- **Lactated ringers is superior to NS**
  - 15-20 cc/kg bolus, then 3 mg/kg/hr (at least 250cc/hr) to **maintain > 0.5 cc/kg/hr urinary output**
  - **Targeted resuscitation by measuring Hct and BUN Q8-12h to ensure adequate fluids.** If BUN is increasing, increase fluids and give 2 L bolus again of crystalloid.
- If US shows gallstone pancreatitis, should get ERCP within 24-48 hours
- Analgesia:
  - IV morphine 2.5-10mg Q 2-6h
  - IV hydromorphone 1-4mg Q3-6h
- If increased triglycerides (>1000), give insulin, heparin, or plasmapheresis (however, most people don't treat this)
- Nutrition:
  - If mild, initiate oral nutrition when pain/nausea allows
  - If severe → NPO, do enteral nutrition with NJ or NG tube (No TPN)
- Antibiotics:
  - **No prophylaxis recommended**
  - If **suspected necrotic pancreatitis, then can give imipenem** 500mg IV Q6-8h (although, most say no antibiotics unless clinical picture worsens after a day or two, or have a tissue diagnosis of infection)
- Debridement of infected necrosis should occur or percutaneous drainage
- ERCP + sphincterectomy reserved for severe cholangitis/sepsis and bili >5, otherwise early ERCP does not decrease risk of complications
- ERCP for bile duct and pancreatic duct lesions
  - Use rectal indomethacin and pancreatic duct stents to prevent post-ERCP pancreatitis
- Zofran
- **If gallstones are the cause, cholecystectomy prior to hospital discharge**

Etiology:

- **Gallstones (30-60%)- most common cause**
- Alcohol (15-30%)- increased if a smoker
- Post ERCP:
  - Occurs in **10-15%** of patients who get an ERCP
  - Use rectal indomethacin and pancreatic duct stents to try to prevent
- Hypertriglyceridemia- >1000, prone to recurrence
- Drugs- see above
- Trauma- blunt abdominal trauma
- Post op
- Uncommon causes:
  - Vasculitis, CT disorders, thrombotic thrombocytopenic purpura, pancreatic cancer, hypercalcemia, pancreas divisum, hereditary pancreatitis, cystic fibrosis, renal failure, infections (mumps, coxsackie, CMV, echovirus), autoimmune, scorpion sting, familial (**PRSS1**, CFTR, SPINK1, CTRC, CASR genes)

Risk Factors:

- Medications
- Alcohol

- Gallstones (female, fat, fertile, flatulent)
- Smoker

Pathogenesis:

- Autodigestion by proteolytic enzymes (trypsinogen, chymotrypsinogen, proelastase, phospholipase A2) are activated in the pancreas acinar cells instead of the gut lumen from **premature activation of trypsin**, which digests pancreatic tissue
- Initial phase- intrapancreatic enzyme activation and acinar injury from trypsin activation, causing acinar injury
- Second phase- activation, chemoattraction, and sequestration of leukocytes and macrophages in the pancreas → inflammatory reaction
- Third phase- effects of activated proteolytic enzymes and cytokines released by inflamed pancreas on distant organs. These digest cell membranes causing proteolysis, edema, interstitial hemorrhage, vascular damage, coagulation necrosis, fat necrosis, and parenchymal cell necrosis

Complications:

- Systemic:
    - Shock
    - **ARDS** (pancreatitis with increasing hypoxemia)
    - AKI
    - GI hemorrhage
    - DIC
- Metabolic:
    - **Hypocalcemia** (poor prognostic marker)
    - Hyperglycemia
    - Increased triglycerides
- Acute fluid collection (30-50%)- no treatment needed
- Pseudocyst (10-20%):
    - Fluid collection that is encapsulated and persists for 4-6 weeks
    - May feel a mass on exam
    - Most resolve spontaneously
    - If >6cm or last >6 weeks → drain with biopsy to rule out cancer
- Sterile pancreatic necrosis (20%):
    - Area of non-viable tissue
    - Do supportive treatment
- Infection (5%):
    - Usually secondary to gram negative rods
    - Infected pancreatic necrosis
    - Pancreatic abscess
    - **Imipenem if necrotizing pancreatitis with worsening clinical picture**
- Ascites or pleural effusion
- Splenic vein thrombosis
- Chronic pancreatitis

Admission Orders:

- Admit to floor if mild, ICU if severe (use prognostic factors)

- Diagnosis acute pancreatitis
- Condition stable, adjust accordingly
- Vital signs Q2h X 3, then Q4h
- Allergies
- Activity up with assistance, bedrest if severe
- Nursing accurate I's/O's, daily weights, assess and treat pain Q2h, call for SBP <100, HR > 110, T > 38.5, increased O2 requirements, or urinary output < 30 ml/h averaged over 4 hours, place NG tube
- Diet NPO
- Fluids LR 15-20 cc/kg bolus, then 3 mg/kg/h (at least 250 cc/hr) to maintain > 0.5 cc/kg/hr urinary output
- Meds:
    - Morphine sulfate IV 1-4 mg Q2h prn pain or hydromorphone
    - Zofran
- Labs/diagnostics:
    - CBC
    - Amylase
    - Lipase
    - CMP
    - Ca2+
    - LDH
    - CRP
    - PT/PTT/INR
    - Abdominal US
    - CT abdomen/pelvis
    - Lipids (fasting)

Discharge Information:

- If mild → when tolerate PO and oral pain meds can go home
- If severe → often stay in hospital for weeks if complications
- If gallstones are the cause → surgical evaluation for cholecystectomy usually before discharge
- If alcohol is the cause → educate about high recurrence, and advise quitting with social worker help

Additional Notes:

-

Acute Kidney Injury

Definitions:

Acute Kidney Injury- abrupt (<48h) increase in Cr ≥ 0.3, increase in Cr ≥ 50%, or urinary output <0.5 mL/kg/h for ≥ 6h

History:

As a provider, you will usually see a high BUN or Cr on labs, which will make you investigate the cause. AKI can range from asymptomatic to severe. It is helpful to know the causes of pre-renal, intrinsic, and post-renal AKI to help you narrow down your history, as the differential of azotemia is vast. Knowing prior Cr levels as a baseline is important.

CC:

HPI:

- COLIDDERRS
- Dehydration?
    - *Pre renal cause*
- Vomiting?
    - *Pre renal cause from volume depletion*
- Diarrhea?
    - *Pre renal cause from volume depletion*
- Polyuria?
    - *Possible post renal obstruction, or pre renal if have CHF*
- Oliguria?
    - *Can be a sign of the AKI, can be from all types of AKI*
- Anuria?
    - *Can be a sign of the AKI, can be from all types of AKI*
- Hematuria?
    - *Can be a sign of intra-renal etiology*
- Recent procedures?
    - *Where? On GU system? Volume depletion?*
- Thirst?
    - *Can be sign of pre renal*
- BPH hx?
    - *Can be sign of post renal cause and needs a foley*
- Straining when urinating?
    - *Can be a sign of BPH and a post renal cause needing a foley*
- Catheter in place?
    - *Can be a sign of neurological disease history and possible post renal cause, and need to make sure foley catheter is working*
- Recent illness?
    - *Can be a sign of dehydration, etc.*
- Fever?
    - *Can be a sign of dehydration*
- Purpura?
    - *Can be a sign of Henoch Schonlein purpura*

- Hemoptysis?
  - *Can be associated with Goodpastures disease*
- Trauma?
- Flank pain?
  - *Can be a sign of kidney stones causing obstruction and post renal cause*
- Suprapubic pain/distension?
  - *Can be a sign of bladder being full and not able to empty requiring a foley*
- Hearing loss?
  - *Can be seen with renal failure in Alports disease*

ROS:

PMH:

- Hx of Kidney disease?
  - *When was it diagnosed?*
  - *How severe (CKD stage?)*
  - *What is your baseline Cr?*
- Hx of BPH?
  - *How severe is it?*
  - *How is it being treated?*
- Chronic indwelling catheter?
  - *Why do you have one?*

Surgical H:

- Any recent procedures?
- GU procedures?

Social H:

- Alcohol, smoking, recreational drugs, job, living situation, sexual history

Family H:

Allergies:

Medications:

Careful medication review is necessary. Many medications can cause AKI, including aminoglycosides, cephalosporins, amphotericin, cisplatin, hydroxyethyl starch solution, beta-lactams, sulfonamides, methotrexate, metformin, NSAIDs, and PPI's amongst others.

Physical Examination:

Assessment of the volume status in patients with AKI is important. Suprapubic examination is necessary in all in case there is bladder distention from bladder overload.

- Vital signs
  - Including orthostatic BP

- Volume status examination
    - Needs to be done, if edema then may need to use diuretics, if dehydrated then may need fluids
- Cardiac exam
    - JVP exam
    - Assess for fluid status and whether they need diuretics or fluids
- Respiratory exam
- Full abdominal exam
    - Enlarged bladder?
    - May need a foley right now
- GU exam, with possible DRE if suspecting BPH
- Edema?
    - Checking for volume status which can change treatment
- Skin turgor?
    - Checking for volume status which can change treatment
- Asterixis?
    - May need to give dialysis
- Skin exam for purpura
    - For Henoch Schonlein purpura
- Hearing evaluation
    - For Alports disease

Differential Diagnosis:

- See symptoms, typical lab values, etiologies, and treatments

Labs:

- UA with culture
    - Nitrates/leukocyte esterase → infection
    - RBCs → hematuria
    - No RBCs but 'positive blood' → rhabdomyolysis (check myoglobin)
    - Eosinophils → acute interstitial nephritis
- Urinary sediment
    - RBC casts → glomerulonephritis
    - WBC casts → pyelonephritis
    - Muddy brown granular casts → acute tubular necrosis
    - Waxy casts → CKD
    - Hyaline → means nothing specific
- BMP
    - Look for electrolyte abnormalities, check for glucose
    - BUN and Cr
- CBC
    - Check for anemia, leukocytosis, etc.
- PT/PTT/INR
    - Late stage CKD can have elevated PT and INR
- BUN:Cr
    - >20:1 → pre-renal
    - <20:1 → intra-renal
- FeNa
    - <1% → pre-renal

- - o >2% → intra-renal
- FeUrea
  - o Can use this in the setting the patient is using diuretics (as FeNa is not as reliable)
  - o <35% → pre-renal
- Urine osmolality
  - o >500 → pre-renal
  - o <350 → intra-renal
- Urinary Na
  - o <20 → pre-renal
  - o >20 → intra-renal
- Urinary specific gravity
  - o >1.018 → pre-renal
- Peripheral smear
  - o Look for schistocytes (HUS/TTP/DIC/pre-eclampsia, antiphospholipid antibody syndrome, malignant hypertension, sclerodermal renal crisis)
- LDH
  - o Possibly DIC, TTP, HUS, pre-eclampsia
- Haptoglobin
  - o Possibly DIC, TTP, HUS, pre-eclampsia
- ANA/ANCA's if suspicious for SLE/Wegners/microscopic polyangiitis/Churg strauss
- Anti-glomerular antibodies if suspecting Good pastures syndrome
- Cryoglobulins if suspecting mixed cryoglobulinemia

Imaging:

- Renal ultrasound and possibly CT
- Post void residual if suspect post renal cause
- Renal biopsy if all other workup fails

Diagnostic Workup:

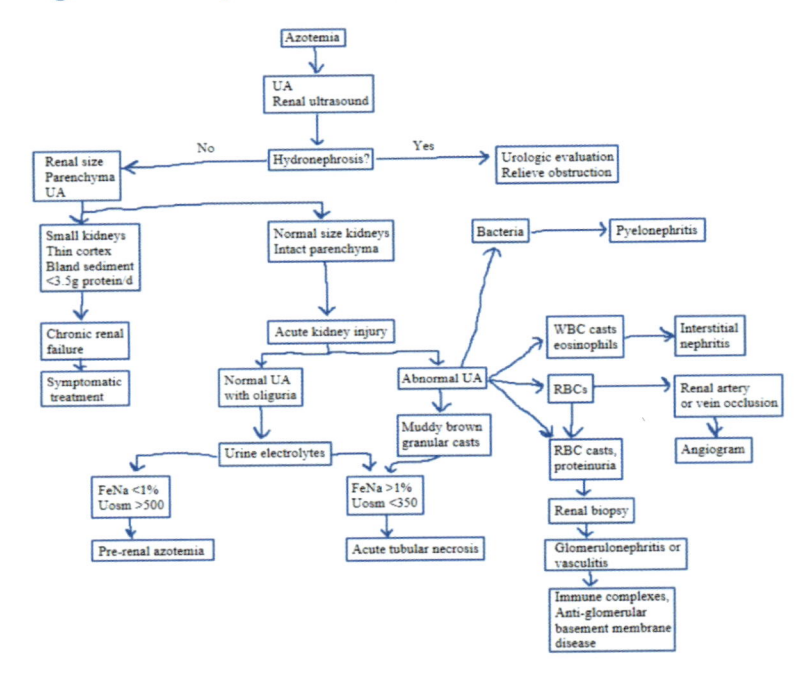

```
                         Azotemia
                            │
                            ▼
                      UA
                      Renal ultrasound
                            │
              No            │           Yes
         ┌──────────── Hydronephrosis? ────────────┐
         │                                          │
         ▼                                          ▼
   Renal size                              Urologic evaluation
   Parenchyma                              Relieve obstruction
   UA
         │
    ┌────┴──────────────────────┐
    ▼                           ▼
Small kidneys            Normal size kidneys          Bacteria ──► Pyelonephritis
Thin cortex              Intact parenchyma               ▲
Bland sediment                  │                        │
<3.5g protein/d                 │                        │
    │                           ▼                                      WBC casts ──► Interstitial
    ▼                     Acute kidney injury                          eosinophils    nephritis
Chronic renal                   │                                          ▲
failure              ┌──────────┴──────────┐                               │
    │                ▼                     ▼                               │
    ▼          Normal UA              Abnormal UA ──────────► RBCs ──► Renal artery
Symptomatic    with oliguria               │                             or vein occlusion
treatment           │                      ▼
                    │               Muddy brown
                    │               granular casts                   RBC casts,      Angiogram
                    ▼                      │                         proteinuria
              Urine electrolytes           │                             │
                    │                      │                             ▼
         ┌──────────┴──────────┐           │                         Renal biopsy
         ▼                     ▼           │                             │
      FeNa <1%             FeNa >1%        │                             ▼
      Uosm >500            Uosm <350       │                     Glomerulonephritis or
         │                     │           │                     vasculitis
         ▼                     ▼           │                             │
   Pre-renal azotemia    Acute tubular necrosis                          ▼
                                                                  Immune complexes,
                                                                  Anti-glomerular
                                                                  basement membrane
                                                                  disease
```

Symptoms, Typical Lab Values, Etiologies, and Treatment:

General Treatment:

- **Bladder foley catheter early**
    - Be wary of how much urine is lost, as you may need to replace that with fluids to prevent dehydration or from actually causing a pre-renal AKI
- Optimize hemodynamics
- Correct fluids and electrolyte imbalances
- Discontinue nephrotoxic medications
- Renal dosing for current medications
- **Are they overloaded, have heart failure, and edema? → give Lasix**
- **Are they septic, borderline shock, and happen to have an elevated Cr? → give fluids**
- **Does the patient have MS (or a neurological disease), a distended, painful bladder, and inability to void? → foley**

Pre-renal AKI:

- Symptoms:
    - Tachycardia
    - Hypotension

- Decreased JVP
- Hx of cirrhosis or heart failure
- Dry mucous membranes
- Typical lab values:
    - **BUN/Cr > 20**
    - FeNa <1%
    - FeUrea <35%
    - Hyaline casts
    - Urinary specific gravity >1.018
    - **Urine osmolality >500 mOsm/kg**
    - **Urinary Na <20**
- Etiologies:
    - **Things that decrease perfusion to the kidneys**
    - Hypovolemia
    - Decreased cardiac output
    - Decreased circulating volume
    - CHF
    - Cirrhosis
    - Venous thromboembolism of renal arteries
    - Renal artery stenosis
    - Hepatorenal syndrome
    - Sepsis
    - NSAIDs
    - ACEI/ARB
    - Cyclosporine
- Treatments:
    - Discontinue medication causing it
    - If blood loss → replace with PRBCs
    - Isotonic crystalloid, or fluid/Na restriction and diuretics depending on fluid status
        - If dry, give IV fluids
        - If wet, give IV lasix
    - Optimize cardiac function

Intrinsic AKI:

- Acute tubular necrosis:
    - Symptoms:
        - Clinical features depend on the cause
    - Typical lab values:
        - **Pigmented granular muddy brown casts**
        - BUN/Cr < 20
        - FeNa >2%
        - ± urinary RBCs and protein from tubular damage
        - **Urinary Na >20**
        - **Urinary osmolality < 350**
    - Etiologies:
        - Drugs (aminoglycosides, amphotericin, cisplatin, methotrexate, hydroxyethyl starch solution)
        - Pigments (hemoglobin, myoglobin)
        - Proteins (Ig light chains, ie multiple myeloma)
        - Crystals (uric acid, acyclovir, methotrexate, indinavir, oral NaPO2, hypercalcemia)
        - Contrast induced kidney injury

- o Treatment:
  - ▪ Removal of offending agent, treat myeloma, treat rhabdomyolysis, treat hyperuricemia
- Acute interstitial nephritis:
  - o Symptoms:
    - ▪ Depends on the cause
    - ▪ Can have a rash
  - o Typical lab values:
    - ▪ WBC's and WBC casts
    - ▪ $\pm$ RBCs with negative urine culture
    - ▪ **+ urine eosinophils if caused by antibiotics**
    - ▪ **+ lymphocytes if caused by NSAIDs**
  - o Etiologies:
    - ▪ Allergic (beta-lactams, sulfonamides, NSAIDs, PPIs)
    - ▪ Infection (pyelonephritis, legionella, TB, leptospirosis)
    - ▪ Infiltrative (sarcoidosis, lymphoma, leukemia)
    - ▪ Autoimmune (Sjogrens, SLE, IgG4)
  - o Treatment:
    - ▪ Remove offending agent
    - ▪ Treat underlying disease
- Small-medium vessel disease:
  - o Symptoms:
    - ▪ Depends on the cause
    - ▪ Purpura in polyarteritis nodosa and Henoch Schonlein purpura
  - o Typical lab values:
    - ▪ $\pm$ RBCs
    - ▪ **+ urine eosinophils in cholesterol emboli**
    - ▪ **Schistocytes in thrombotic microangiopathies** (HUS/TTP/DIC/pre-eclampsia, antiphospholipid antibody syndrome, malignant hypertension, sclerodermal renal crisis)
  - o Etiologies:
    - ▪ Cholesterol emboli
    - ▪ Polyarteritis nodosa
    - ▪ Thrombotic microangiopathies (HUS/TTP/DIC/pre-eclampsia, antiphospholipid antibody syndrome, malignant hypertension, sclerodermal renal crisis)
  - o Treatment:
    - ▪ Treat the underlying cause
- Glomerulonephritis:
  - o Many causes and different treatments

Post-renal AKI:

- **Foley catheter**
- **Things that cause obstruction of the urinary system**
- Bladder neck:
  - o BPH, prostate cancer, neurogenic bladder
  - o Use anticholinergics and treat cancer
- Ureteral:
  - o Must affect both ureters

- Malignancy, lymphadenopathy, retroperitoneal, fibrosis, nephrolithiasis
- Treat with catheter, stop anticholinergics

Miscellaneous Complications and Their Treatments:

- Malnutrition- 20-30 kcal/kg/day, protein is 0.8-1.0 g/kg/day
- Anemia- if uremic bleeding use desmopressin or estrogen
- GI prophylaxis- with Pepcid or protonix
- DVT prophylaxis- don't use LMWH or Xa inhibitors
- Rhabdomyolysis- aggressive fluids
- Tumor lysis syndrome- aggressive fluids + allopurinol or rasbiscurase, possibly dialysis
- Hyponatremia- restrict free water
- Hyperkalemia- restrict dietary K+, stop K+ sparing diuretics (ACEIs, ARBs, spironolactone), stop NSAIDs, give loop inhibitors, give insulin + glucose, give inhaled beta-2 agonists, **give calcium gluconate if EKG changes are present**
- Metabolic acidosis- NaHCO3-
- Hyperphosphatemia- decrease dietary phosphate, give calcium acetate
- Hypocalcemia- if symptomatic give calcium carbonate or calcium gluconate
- Hypermagnesia- stop Mg containing antacids
- Hyperuricemia- no treatment unless tumor lysis syndrome then fluids and allopurinol

Dialysis Indications:

- **AEIOU:**
    - **A**cidosis- pH < 7.1
    - **E**lectrolyte disorder- hyperkalemia (>6.5 or rapidly increasing, tumor lysis syndrome)
    - **I**ntoxication- methanol, ethylene glycol, lithium, salicyclates
    - **O**verload, volume which is refractory to diuretics
    - **U**remia- pericarditis, encephalopathy, bleeding

Risk Factors:

- Older age
- CKD
- Chronic HTN
- Diabetes
- BPH
- Prostate cancer
- Chronic NSAID use

Pathogenesis:

- Depends on what is causing it

Complications:

- Uremia

- Hypo/hypervolemia
- Hyponatremia
- Hyperkalemia
    - If have hypokalemia yet have an AKI, suspect a renal tubular acidosis syndrome where you are not able to retain K+
- Anion gap metabolic acidosis
- Hyperphosphatemia
- Hypocalcemia
- Bleeding
- Infections
- Malnutrition

Admission Orders:

- Admit to floor, or telemetry if have hyperkalemia
- Diagnosis acute kidney injury
- Condition guarded
- Vital signs routine, check orthostatics on admission and once per shift
- Allergies
- Activity ad lib
- Nursing place foley, strict I's/O's, daily weights, call for urinary output <200 mL/shift or SaO2 <92%
- Diet renal (low Na, low K, low P)
- Fluids NS 250 ml/h X 3h, then reassess, or fluid restriction depending on volume status
- Meds:
    - Pepcid
    - Heparin
    - Discontinue nephrotoxic medications
- Labs/diagnostics:
    - UA with microscopy
    - CBC
    - CMP
    - Ca2+
    - Mg
    - Phosphate
    - FeNa
    - Urinary Na
    - Urinary osmolality
    - Urinary specific gravity
    - Urinary sediment
    - PT/PTT/INR
    - Renal ultrasound

Discharge Information:

- Depends on the diagnosis
- Pre-renal with volume depletion stay usually 2-3 days
- Acute tubular necrosis → dialysis for 1-3 weeks
- Follow renal diet and daily weights, call PCP if gain more than 3-4 lbs in a day

Additional Notes:

-

Chronic Kidney Disease

Definitions:

<u>Chronic kidney disease-</u> spectrum of different processes associated with abnormal kidney function and decline in GFR

Stage	Description	GFR
1	Kidney Damage with normal GFR	≥ 90
2	Kidney damage with mild GFR	60-89
3A	Mild to moderate GFR	45-59
3B	Moderate GFR	30-45
4	Severe GFR	15-30
5	Kidney failure	<15 or dialysis

History:

The history in someone with chronic kidney disease is mostly to assess for risk factors that leads to loss of kidney function. Certain precipitants can invoke an acute on chronic kidney injury, leading to hospitalizations. It's important to also know about what type of treatment they are receiving, and if they are receiving dialysis, how often, and if they are compliant.

CC:

HPI:

- COLIDDERRS
    - *Generally a person with history of kidney disease and with gradual symptoms of uremia (anorexia, n/v, uremic pericarditis, delirium, seizures, coma) in decompensated states*
- Change in mental status?
    - *Sign of possibly uremia and potential need for dialysis*
- Appetite changes?
    - *Commonly get anorexia*
- Weight loss?
    - *Commonly get anorexia and cachectic*
- N/V?
    - *Common sign as toxins buildup that usually would be cleared by kidneys*
- Palpitations?
    - *Can cause fatal arrhythmias as K+ buildsup*
- SOB?
    - *From fluid buildup, diurese first, then do dialysis if no help*
- Hiccups?
    - *Symptom of uremia from neuromuscular abnormalities*
- Cramps?
    - *Symptom of uremia from neuromuscular abnormalities and electrolyte abnormalities*

- Pruritus?
    - *Deposition of urochromes in the skin, sign of uremia*
- Restless legs?
    - *Neuromuscular abnormalities from electrolyte imbalances and vascular disease*
- Oliguria?
    - *Common in CKD*
- Skin ulcers?
    - *Sign of calciphylaxis*

ROS:

PMH:

- Hx of HTN?
    - *Can damage the kidneys overtime causing the CKD*
    - *How severe?*
    - *How is it being treated?*
- Hx of Diabetes?
    - *Most common cause of CKD*
    - *How severe?*
    - *How is it being treated?*
- Hx of Cancer?

Surgical H:

Social H:

- Alcohol, smoking, recreational drugs, job, living situation, sexual history

Family H:

- Hx of CKD?
    - Alports (hearing issues), Fabrys disease, Cystinosis

Allergies:

Medications:

- NSAIDs
- Antibiotics (especially aminoglycosides and cephalosporins)
- Chemotherapy drugs
- Anti-retrovirals
- PPIs

Physical Examination:

The physical exam is used to look for complications that can occur with CKD and ESRD. End organ damage from HTN should be assessed. If the patient is altered you should look for asterixis and a pericardial friction rub as uremia can occur.

- BP

- - Hypertension common from salt and water retention and increased renin-angiotension-aldosterone system activation
- Fundoscopy if able to perform
    - Looking for papilledema
- LV heave
    - Sign of heart failure due to volume overload from CKD
- S4
    - Sign of heart failure due to volume overload from CKD
- Edema
    - Very common and need to diurese or perform dialysis
- Sensory polyneuropathy
    - Common in CKD, especially if diabetic
- Palpate kidneys
    - See if they have polycystic kidney disease
- Asterixis
    - Look for uremia
- Pericardial friction rub
    - Looks for uremia from uremic pericarditis

Differential Diagnosis:

- See etiology

Labs:

- **Previous BUN and Cr**
    - Very important to determine where they were and how they compare to that now
- GFR
    - For staging their CKD (see table above)
- Urinary albumin
    - Part of staging
- CBC
    - Look for anemia (normocytic normochromic), leukocytosis
- CMP
    - Look for electrolyte abnormalities, especially K+, glucose, LFTs
- If age >35 and unexplained CKD, get serum and urine protein electrophoresis to look for multiple myeloma
- Vit D
    - Usually low in CKD
- Ca
    - Can be hypocalcemia from increased phosphate retention or increased calcium
- Mg
- PTH
    - Can be increased in CKD (secondary hyperparathyroidism from decreased calcium because phosphate is increased and binds to calcium to decrease it)
- Alkaline phosphatase
    - Can be increased in secondary hyperparathyroidism from bone turnover due to increased PTH
- UA

- Waxy casts can show CKD
- Protein:Cr or 24h urine protein collection, as well as urine microalbumin
    - See how much protein is being lost in a day

Imaging:

- Renal ultrasound- **most useful** (size, symmetry, masses, obstruction, scarring)
    - Shrunken kidneys is a sign of CKD
- Doppler sonography
    - Assess blood flow to the kidneys
- CT or MRI for renovascular disease (if kidneys are not the same size)
    - Checking for renal artery stenosis or fibromuscular dysplasia
- Voiding cystogram if suspect reflux nephropathy
- No contrast studies, avoid IV dye
- Biopsy- NOT advised with bilaterally small kidneys because of scarring
    - Contraindicated if uncontrolled HTN, active UTI, bleeding diathesis, and severe obesity

Diagnosis of CKD:

- Most important is to distinguish newly diagnosed CKD from acute or subacute renal failure
- Previous Cr levels are very helpful
- Normal Cr values from recent months or even years could be more subacute and hence possibly reversible
- If history suggests multiple systemic symptoms of recent onset, it should be assumed it's not chronic but part of the illness
- Renal biopsy can be performed if early (stage 1-3) but not always indicated (ie a history of diabetes for 15-20 years with retinopathy and nephrotic range proteinuria and absence of hematuria, then biopsy is not necessary)
- In absence of clinical diagnosis, renal biopsy may be needed
- Ultrasound showing small, scarred kidneys

Treatment:

- Optimize glucose control in diabetes
    - Goal A1c <7.0
- Immunosuppressive agents for glomerulonephritis
- Serial GFRs
    - To keep up with stage of CKD or see if treatment is working
- Keep BP controlled, **goal <140/90**, to keep proteinuria at a minimum
    - **ACEI/ARBs** → constrict the efferent arterioles and slow the progress of disease in both diabetes and non-diabetic CKD
    - **Benazepril in Severe CKD trial (2006, NEJM)-** Benazepril slows renal disease progression in patients with stage 4 non-diabetic CKD when compared to placebo
- Combination of an ACEI and ARB has a greater reduction on proteinuria compared to either agent alone
    - This increases the risk of AKI and cardiac events however
- Diltiazem or verapamil if ACEI intolerant
- Adjusting doses of renally excreted drugs

- Avoid radiocontrast agents and gadollium
- Protein restriction if signs of uremia impending (anorexia, n/v, pruritus)
- Renal replacement therapy indications:
    - Uremic pericarditis, encephalopathy, intractable muscle cramping, anorexia, nausea not attributable to PUD, malnutrition, fluid/electrolyte imbalances (hyperkalemia and fluid overload)
- Dialysis, hopefully started before onset of severe symptoms/uremia → increases survival
    - **IDEAL trial (2010, NEJM)-** In patients with stage V CKD, there was no difference in survival or clinical outcomes between early or late initiation of dialysis. This trial supports current practice guidelines that dialysis should be initiated in symptomatic patients due to uremia or in asymptomatic patients with an extremely low GFR, approximately 10.
- Pt education
- Kidney transplant

Etiology:

- **Diabetes- most common cause**
- HTN associated CKD
- Glomerulonephritis
- Autosomal dominant polycystic kidney disease (ADPKD)
- Other cystic and tubulointerstital nephropathies

Risk Factors:

- Small for gestational age birth weight
- Childhood obesity
- HTN
- Diabetes
- Autoimmune disease
- Age
- African Americans
- Family Hx of CKD
- Previous Hx of AKI
- Presence of proteinuria
- Abnormal urinary sediment
- Structural abnormality of urinary tract
- ADPKD

Pathogenesis:

- Chronic kidney disease:
    - Initiating mechanism of underlying disease
    - Progressive hyperfiltration and hypertrophy of viable nephrons
    - **Increase in RAAS**, increased cytokines, eventually sclerosis
- Uremic syndrome:
    - Accumulation of urea and Cr does **NOT** account for the many symptoms and signs of uremia
    - Three spheres of dysfunction:

- Consequences of accumulated toxins
- Loss of kidney function causing fluid/electrolyte/hormone regulation dysfunction
- Systemic inflammation and its vascular and nutritional consequences
  - Consequences of accumulated toxins:
    - Water soluble hydrophobic, protein-bound, charged/uncharged compounds accumulate
    - Products of amino acid and nucleic acid metabolites accumulate
  - Loss of kidney function causing fluid/electrolyte/hormone regulation dysfunction:
    - Anemia, malnutrition, abnormal metabolism, PTH/VitD/sex hormones/FGF-2/insulin/steroid hormones/prolactin levels change
  - Systemic inflammation and its vascular and nutritional consequences:
    - Inflammation → malnutrition
    - Inflammation → atherosclerosis/calcification syndrome
    - This accelerates vascular disease

Clinical/Lab/Complications of CKD and Their Treatment:

Fluid, electrolyte, and acid base disorders:

- Total Na and water is increased:
  - Edema
  - Treatment:
    - Salt restriction
    - Loop diuretics
    - Add metolazone if GFR < 30 and have ECF volume expansion
- Hyperkalemia:
  - **Fatal arrhythmias**
    - Peaked T waves, widened QRS, widened PR interval, widened QT, torsades
  - Treatment:
    - Dietary decrease of K+
    - May need **calcium gluconate if EKG changes are present**
    - Insulin with glucose
    - Beta 2 agonists
    - Loop diuretics, dialysis
    - NOT Kayxeylate for acute (risk of bowel necrosis)
- Metabolic acidosis:
  - Decreased ammonia production in kidneys → decreased excretion of protons
  - **Anion gap metabolic acidosis**
  - Treatment:
    - Sodium bicarbonate

Calcium/Phosphate disorders:

- Bone manifestations:
    - Secondary hyperparathyroidism with increased PTH → **Osteitis fibrosa cystica** (renal osteodystrophy)
    - Decreased calcium with increased phosphate
        - Phosphate cannot be excreted from the kidney, which then binds to and decreases calcium
    - Increased alkaline phosphatase from bone turnover from increased PTH
    - Treatment:
        - Prevention
        - Use low phosphate diet
        - Calcium acetate (phosphate binder)
        - Sevalemer or lanthanum
        - Calcitriol
        - Cinalcet (increases calcium receptor sensitivity → decreases PTH secretion)
- Increased cardiovascular mortality:
    - Increased vascular calcification of CAD
- Calciphylaxis:
    - Especially if on warfarin

Cardiovascular abnormalities:

- **Leading cause of morbidity and mortality in all CKD patients**
- General treatment:
    - BP < 140/90 with ACEI/ARBs
    - Salt restriction
    - Lifestyle changes
    - Statins
- Ischemic vascular disease:
    - Occlusive coronary, CVA, PVD, HTN, dyslipidemia, hyperhomocystinemia
    - Cardiac troponins are elevated in CKD without evidence of acute ischemia
- Heart failure:
    - Secondary to ischemia, LVH, cardiomyopathy, salt and water retention
    - Pulmonary edema can occur, SOB with "bat wing" distribution of alveolar edema fluid on CXR
- Pericardial disease:
    - Chest pain with respirations, friction rub
    - P-R depression and diffuse ST elevation, pericardial effusion
    - Treatment:
        - If uremic → dialysis
        - Pericardial drainage if tamponade

Hematologic abnormalities:

- Normocytic normochromic anemia:
    - Comes from **decreased erythropoietin production from kidneys**
    - Fatigue, increased cardiac output, can lead to heart failure

- Treatment:
  - Iron supplements
  - Rarely EPO
  - Only do Hgb to 10-11.5 → higher has an increased mortality
  - **TREAT trial (2009, NEJM)**- TREAT demonstrated that targeting a hemoglobin of > 13 with erythrocyte-stimulating agents does not confer a survival benefit in T2DM with CKD, but does increase the risk of stroke

- Abnormal hemostasis:
  - Increased bleeding time, decreased activity of platelet factor III
  - Abnormal platelet aggregation and adhesiveness and impaired prothrombin consumption **(platelet dysfunction)**
  - Bruising, bleeding, menorrhagia, GI bleed, proteinuria
  - **Loss of antithrombin III → hypercoagulable state**
  - Treatment:
    - Desmopressin
    - Cryoprecipitate
    - IV conjugated estrogens
    - Transfusions
    - EPO
    - Avoid LMWH (lovenox) and Xa inhibitors

Neuromuscular abnormalities:

- CNS, peripheral, and autonomic neuropathies
- Muscle function abnormalities
- Memory/concentration/sleep disturbances
- Hiccups, cramps, twitching, asterixis, seizures, comas, restless leg syndrome
- Treatment:
  - For peripheral neuropathy not explained by another cause, do renal replacement therapy

GI and nutritional abnormalities:

- Uremic fetor (urine breath) → dysguesia
- Gastritis, PUD, abdominal pain, n/v, GI bleed
- Malnutrition
- Treatment:
  - Protein restriction, which can even treat the n/v

Endocrine-metabolic disturbances:

- Glucose metabolism impaired → hyperglycemia
- Estrogen low in women → menstrual abnormalities, infertility, osteoporosis, heart disease risk
- Decreased testosterone in men → sexual dysfunction and oligospermia

Dermatologic abnormalities:

- Pruritus:
  - Deposition of urochromes

- o Treatment:
    - Treat hyperphosphatemia, local moisturizers, topical glucocorticoids, PO anthistamines, UV radiation, cholestyramine, capsaicin cream
- Nephrogenic fibrosing dermatopathy:
    - o Subcutaneous induration
- Calciphylaxis

Additional Notes:

- Important clinical trials:
    - o **Benazepril in Severe CKD trial (2006, NEJM)-** Benazepril slows renal disease progression in patients with stage 4 non-diabetic CKD when compared to placebo
    - o **TREAT trial (2009, NEJM)-** TREAT demonstrated that targeting a hemoglobin of > 13 with erythrocyte-stimulating agents does not confer a survival benefit in T2DM with CKD, but does increase the risk of stroke
    - o **IDEAL trial (2010, NEJM)-** In patients with stage V CKD, there was no difference in survival or clinical outcomes between early or late initiation of dialysis. This trial supports current practice guidelines that dialysis should be initiated in symptomatic patients due to uremia or in asymptomatic patients with an extremely low GFR, approximately 10.
- GFR based diuretic therapy:
    - o GFR ≥ 30 → thiazides
    - o GFR < 30 → loops 1-2X daily
    - o GFR < 30 and ECF volume expansion → loop + thiazide

Hyponatremia

Definitions:

Hyponatremia- serum sodium <136, most often due to excess water relative to sodium

Hypertonic hyponatremia- hyponatremia with plasma osmolality >295

Hypotonic hyponatremia- hyponatremia with plasma osmolality <275

History:

Hyponatremia is usually found on screening labs. It is important to know if this is acute or chronic, how severe symptoms are, and to know if the patient has risks for neurological complications (alcoholism, malnourishment, cirrhosis, hypoxia, hypokalemia). Symptoms can be nonspecific, but knowing whether the patient has symptomatic hyponatremia will change level of care and the initial treatment approach. Volume status can be difficult to assess, but is important to help determine the cause and workup. Medication review is also essential.

CC:

HPI:

- COLIDDERRS
- Headache?
- Nausea/vomiting?
- Confusion?
- Seizures?
- Obtundation?

ROS:

PMH:

- Hx of Heart failure?
    - *Common cause of hypervolemic hyponatremia*
- Hx of Cirrhosis?
    - *Common cause of hypervolemic hyponatremia*
- Hx of Kidney disease?
    - *Common cause of hypervolemic hyponatremia*
- Hx of Hypothyroidism?
    - *Can cause hyponatremia*
- Hx of Adrenal insufficiency?
    - *Can cause hyponatremia*

Surgical H:

Social H:

- **Alcohol**, smoking, recreational drugs, job, living situation, sexual history
    - Beer potomania causes hyponatremia

Family H:

Allergies:

Medications:

- There are many different medications that can cause hyponatremia
- Diuretics (especially thiazides), SSRIs, TCAs, NSAIDs, carbamazepine, vinctristine, antipsychotic drugs, AVP analogues, desmopressin, oxytocin, vasopressin, chlorpropamide, clofibrate, nicotine, narcotics, cyclophosphamide, etc.

Physical Examination:

Once hyponatremia has been established, it is important to assess the fluid status of the patient. This can be difficult. Look at vitals, orthostatics, JVP, skin turgor, mucous membranes, and peripheral edema. Assess mental status thoroughly.

- Vital signs
    - Tachycardia and hypotension suggest hypovolemia, hypoxia
- Assess mental status
    - Confusion, obtundation can be signs of severe symptomatic hyponatremia
- Neurologic exam
    - Focal neuro signs can be present
- Edema
- Skin turgor
- Mucous membranes

Differential Diagnosis:

- See etiology

Labs and Approach to Hypotonic Hyponatremia:

- Plasma osmolality
    - First step in hyponatremia evaluation
    - Normal is 275-295 mOsm
    - If elevated, look into hyperglycemia, mannitol, sucrose
    - If isotonic, usually from hyperlipidemia or hyperproteinemia
    - If hypotonic, have to assess volume status and measure urine osmolality and urine Na levels
- Urine osmolality
    - If patients plasma osmolality is hypotonic then measure urine osmolality
    - If urine osmolality is <100 mOsm, this is consistent with appropriately suppressed ADH release (primary polydipsia or decreased solute intake)

- If urine osmolality is >100 mOsm, this is consistent with inappropriately increased ADH levels and volume status is the next step
- Urinary Na
  - Helps to determine the cause of hypotonic hyponatremia (see flow chart below)
- TSH
- AM cortisol, ACTH stimulation test if indicated
- HIV Ab

Approach to hypotonic hyponatremia:

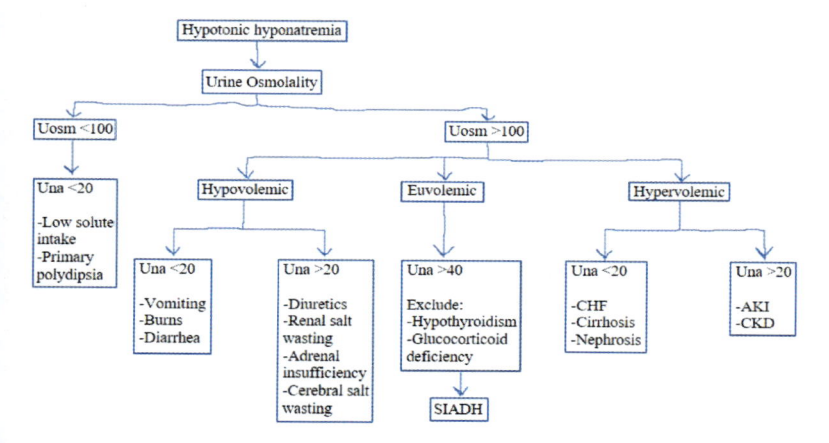

```
                    Hypotonic hyponatremia
                             ↓
                     Urine Osmolality
              ↙                           ↘
       Uosm <100                         Uosm >100
          ↓                    ↙            ↓           ↘
    Una <20            Hypovolemic      Euvolemic    Hypervolemic
   -Low solute              ↓              ↓              ↓
    intake            ↙         ↘          ↓         ↙         ↘
   -Primary      Una <20      Una >20   Una >40   Una <20    Una >20
   polydipsia   -Vomiting   -Diuretics  Exclude:  -CHF       -AKI
                -Burns      -Renal salt -Hypothy- -Cirrhosis -CKD
                -Diarrhea    wasting     roidism  -Nephrosis
                            -Adrenal    -Glucocor-
                             insuffi-    ticoid
                             ciency      deficiency
                            -Cerebral        ↓
                             salt         SIADH
                             wasting
```

Etiology and Treatment:

Acute symptomatic hyponatremia:

- These patients need to be treated in the ICU if the symptoms are severe (seizures, obtundation, whereas patients with headache, mild confusion, can generally be treated on the floor and do not need hypertonic saline)
- Hypertonic saline with goal increase in Na of 4-6 mEq in the first 4 hours and maintenance of that for 24 hours (to avoid osmotic demyelination syndrome)
  - Maintenance fluids with 3% NS at rate of 30 cc/hr
  - Can bolus the patient with 3% NS 100mL over 30 minutes instead
  - Q2h Na and neuro checks
  - If not at goal, can consider another 100mL bolus of 3% NS

Asymptomatic hyponatremia:

- Hypertonic hyponatremia:
  - Hyperglycemia from DKA or hyperosmolar hyperglycemic state, mannitol, sucrose
  - Treat the underlying cause
- Hypotonic hyponatremia with urine osmolality <100:
  - Primary polydipsia or decreased solute intake

- Correct underlying cause
- Hypovolemic hypotonic hyponatremia:
    - Urinary Na <20:
        - Extra-renal losses from vomiting, diarrhea, burns, pancreatitis
        - Treat the underlying cause
        - Maintenance IVFs with NS to suppress circulating ADH and induce water diuresis
    - Urinary Na >20:
        - Diuretic therapy, renal salt wasting, adrenal insufficiency, cerebral salt wasting
        - Treat the underlying cause
        - Maintenance IVFs with NS to suppress circulating ADH and induce water diuresis
- Euvolemic hypotonic hyponatremia:
    - Urinary Na is usually >40
    - Hypothyroidism, adrenal insufficiency, SIADH
    - Exclude hypothyroidism and adrenal insufficiency before doing a workup for SIADH
    - Treat underlying cause
        - Usually free water restrict these patients, can try diuresis with lasix
    - SIADH causes:
        - Malignancy- Lung, brain, GI, GU, lymphoma, leukemia, thymoma, mesothelioma
        - Pulmonary- pneumonia, TB, aspergillosis, asthma, COPD, pneumothorax
        - Intracranial- trauma, stroke, hemorrhage, infection, hydrocephalus, Guillan-Barre syndrome
        - Drugs- Diuretics (especially thiazides), SSRIs, TCAs, NSAIDs, carbamazepine, vinctristine, antipsychotic drugs, AVP analogues, desmopressin, oxytocin, vasopressin, chlorpropamide, clofibrate, nicotine, narcotics, cyclophosphamide, etc.
        - Infections- HIV, RMSF
- Hypervolemic hypotonic hyponatremia:
    - Urinary Na <20:
        - Chronic heart failure, cirrhosis, nephrosis
        - Fluid and Na restriction
        - Diuretic therapy
        - ACEI if due to heart failure
        - If hyponatremia is resistant to above measures in a patient with heart failure, consider tolvaptan
        - If considering nephrosis, renal consult
    - Urinary Na >20:
        - Acute or chronic kidney failure
        - Fluid and Na restriction
        - Diuretic therapy
        - Renal consult

Risk Factors:

- Medications (as above)

- Poor oral intake or diet (tea and toast diet)
- Alcoholism (beer potomania)
- Psychiatric history
- Elderly

Complications:

- Cerebral edema
- Brain herniation
- Cardiopulmonary arrest
- Seizure
- Coma
- Death
- **Osmotic demyelination syndrome:**
    - Chronic hyponatremia is associated with the loss of osmotically active organic osmolytes from astrocytes which provide protection against brain cell swelling
    - As you correct Na back into the circulation, water will be pulled out of these cells, causing brain volume to decrease, resulting in demyelination of brain cells, and leads to apoptosis of these cells
    - Patients with chronic hyponatremia and lower Na on presentation are more at risk with too rapid of Na correction
    - If overcorrection occurs, give D5W at ~150 mL/hr and give desmopressin 2mcg IV Q6h with Q2h Na checks

Admission Orders:

- Admit to floor/ICU
- Diagnosis hyponatremia
- Condition stable/guarded/critical
- Vital signs routine, orthostatics Q4h
- Allergies
- Activity as tolerated
- Nursing call for hypoxia, seizures, obtundation
- Diet Na restriction and fluid restriction if indicated
- Fluids NS, hypertonic saline, or fluid restriction depending on clinical context
- Meds:
    - Depends on cause
    - Diuretics if hypervolemic
- Labs/diagnostics:
    - BMP
    - Q2h Na checks
    - Plasma osmolality
    - Urine osmolality
    - Urine Na
    - TSH
    - AM cortisol
    - ACTH stimulation test
    - HIV Ab

Additional Notes:

-

Anemia

Definitions:

Anemia- decrease in RBC mass: Hct <41% or Hgb <13.5 (men); Hct <36% or Hgb <12 (women)

History:

Anemia is usually first noted in screening laboratory tests. It mostly presents with very nonspecific symptoms, or none at all. You have to think of reasons why someone would be anemic once it is seen on CBC to find out from the history what is causing it.

CC:

HPI:

- COLIDDERRS
    - *Can be asymptomatic, classic symptoms are fatigue, headache, poor concentration, nausea, vague abdominal discomfort, SOB*
- Fatigue?
    - *Common symptom of anemia*
- DOE?
    - *Might not be able to get enough oxygen to tissues and heart when exercising*
- Chest pain?
    - *Possibly low oxygen delivery to the heart*
- Bleeding (stool, urine, mouth, etc)?
    - *Possible acute source of the anemia*
- Recent illness?
    - *Many illnesses can cause anemia, such as mycoplasma pneumoniae, mononucleosis, etc.*
- Drugs?
    - See below
- Alcohol?
    - *Possible B12/folate deficiency and macrocytic anemia*
- Diet (PICA)?
    - *Sign of iron deficiency anemia*
- Fever?
    - *Possible sign of infection induced anemia*
- Weight loss?
    - *Can be a sign of colon cancer with anemia or any malignancy*
- Night sweats?
    - *Can be a sign of cancer anemia*
- Petechiae?

ROS:

PMH:

- Hx of Anemia?
    - *What has been done for it in the past*

Surgical H:

Social H:

- Alcohol, smoking, recreational drugs, job, living situation, sexual history
- Geographic background (ie middle eastern/African American for G6PD, alpha thalassemia, and hereditary spherocytosis)
- Diet (PICA)

Family H:

- Fm Hx of anemia?
    - *Was a diagnosis made that is genetic?*

Allergies:

Medications:

- Antibiotics- cephalosporins, sulfonamides, rifampin, ribavirin
- Cardiovascular- methyldopa, procainamide, quinidine, thiazides
- TCAs, phenothiazines, NSAIDs, sulfonylureas, methotrexate, 5-FU, rasbiscurase
- G6PD deficiency- sulfonamides, dapsone, primaquine, doxorubicin, methylene blue

Physical Examination:

There is a wide variety of physical exam findings in anemia that could be present based on the cause of the anemia. It could range from minor abnormalities in the skin, to neurologic symptoms. It's important to keep in the back of your head the etiologies of anemia and what their physical exam findings may be.

- VS
    - Tachycardia, orthostatic hypotension
- Pale (mucous membranes, palmar creases)
- Forceful heartbeat, possible flow murmur
- Jaundice (in hemolytic anemias)
- Splenomegaly (thalassemia, hereditary spherocytosis, chronic hemolysis, myelofibrosis)
- Petechiae/purpura (bleeding disorder)
- Glossitis (Fe, folate, B12 deficiency)
- Koilonychia (Fe deficiency)
- Neurologic abnormalities (B12 deficiency)

Differential Diagnosis:

- See etiology

Labs:

- CBC
  - Hgb, Hct, MCV, MCH, MCHC, plt
- Reticulocyte index
  - ≥2.5 → hemolytic anemia or blood loss
  - <2.5 → non-hemolytic anemia
- Iron studies
  - Serum Fe, TIBC, TIBC sat %, ferritin
- Peripheral blood smear for morphology
  - Look for schistocytes, macrocytes, hypersegmented neutrophils, sickled RBCs, etc.
- LDH
  - Increased in hemolytic anemia
- Haptoglobin
  - Decreased in hemolytic anemia
- Indirect bilirubin
  - Increased in hemolytic anemias
- Bone marrow aspirate/biopsy
  - Reserved for when a diagnosis isn't clear

Etiology, Pathogenesis, and Treatment:

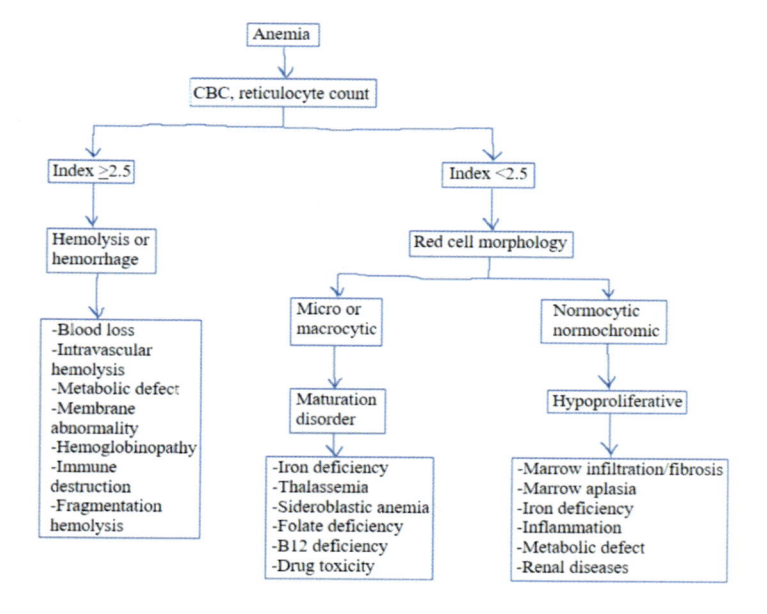

```
                    Anemia
                      ↓
            CBC, reticulocyte count
              ↓                    ↓
        Index ≥2.5            Index <2.5
              ↓                    ↓
        Hemolysis or      Red cell morphology
        hemorrhage          ↓           ↓
              ↓        Micro or    Normocytic
                       macrocytic  normochromic
                          ↓             ↓
                      Maturation   Hypoproliferative
                      disorder
```

Index ≥2.5 → Hemolysis or hemorrhage:
- Blood loss
- Intravascular hemolysis
- Metabolic defect
- Membrane abnormality
- Hemoglobinopathy
- Immune destruction
- Fragmentation hemolysis

Maturation disorder:
- Iron deficiency
- Thalassemia
- Sideroblastic anemia
- Folate deficiency
- B12 deficiency
- Drug toxicity

Hypoproliferative:
- Marrow infiltration/fibrosis
- Marrow aplasia
- Iron deficiency
- Inflammation
- Metabolic defect
- Renal diseases

Microcytic:

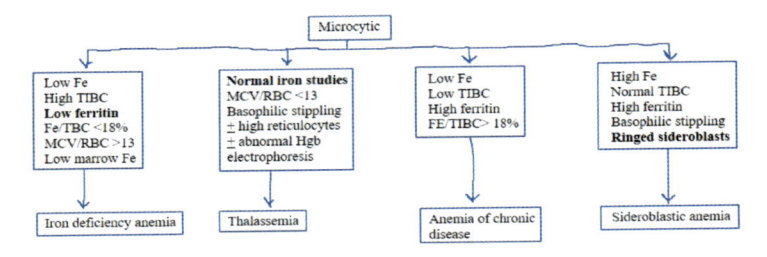

```
                            ┌─────────────┐
                            │  Microcytic │
                            └─────────────┘
         ┌──────────────┬──────────┴──────────┬──────────────┐
         ▼              ▼                     ▼              ▼
┌─────────────┐ ┌─────────────────┐ ┌──────────────┐ ┌────────────────┐
│ Low Fe      │ │ Normal iron     │ │ Low Fe       │ │ High Fe        │
│ High TIBC   │ │ studies         │ │ Low TIBC     │ │ Normal TIBC    │
│ Low ferritin│ │ MCV/RBC <13     │ │ High ferritin│ │ High ferritin  │
│ Fe/TBC <18% │ │ Basophilic      │ │ FE/TIBC> 18% │ │ Basophilic     │
│ MCV/RBC >13 │ │ stippling       │ │              │ │ stippling      │
│ Low marrow  │ │ ± high          │ │              │ │ Ringed         │
│ Fe          │ │ reticulocytes   │ │              │ │ sideroblasts   │
│             │ │ ± abnormal Hgb  │ │              │ │                │
│             │ │ electrophoresis │ │              │ │                │
└─────────────┘ └─────────────────┘ └──────────────┘ └────────────────┘
       ▼                ▼                   ▼                ▼
┌──────────────┐  ┌────────────┐    ┌──────────────┐  ┌────────────────┐
│ Iron         │  │ Thalassemia│    │ Anemia of    │  │ Sideroblastic  │
│ deficiency   │  │            │    │ chronic      │  │ anemia         │
│ anemia       │  │            │    │ disease      │  │                │
└──────────────┘  └────────────┘    └──────────────┘  └────────────────┘
```

- Iron deficiency anemia:
    - Decreased marrow Fe and depleted body Fe → decreased heme synthesis → microcytes → anemia
    - Angular cheilosis, atrophic glossitis, PICA
    - Nail spooning (koilonychia)
    - **Decreased ferritin** and iron, increased TIBC
    - Etiologies:
        - Chronic bleeding (eg colon cancer)
        - Decreased supply (eg malnutrition, Celiacs, Crohns)
        - Increased demand (eg pregnancy)
    - Treatment:
        - Oral Fe (Ferrous sulfate 325 PO TID X 3-6 months)
- Thalassemias:
    - Decrease synthesis of alpha or beta globin chains of Hgb → don't make correct subunits → destruction of RBCs and erythroid precursors, therefore anemia from hemolysis and ineffective erythropoiesis
    - Alpha thalassemia → 3,2,1,0 traits
    - Beta thalassemia → 1 or 2 mutations
    - Chipmunk facies, crew cut appearance on X-ray, fractures, hepatosplenomegaly (**extramedullary hematopoiesis**), high-output CHF, bilirubin gallstones, chronic transfusions
    - MCV < 70, **normal Fe studies**, ± abnormal Hgb electrophoresis
    - Treatment:
        - Folate
        - Transfusions- deferoxamine or deferasirox (PO)
        - Splenectomy if transfusion increase ≥ 50%
- Inflammatory anemia (anemia of chronic disease):
    - Decreased RBC production from impaired Fe utilization and functional Fe deficiency from **increased hepcidin**
    - Autoimmune disorders, chronic infection, inflammation, HIV, malignancy, CKD
    - Decreased Fe, **decreased TIBC**, ± **increased ferritin**, can be normocytic
    - Treatment:
        - Treat underlying disease ± Fe and/or EPO
        - Fe if ferritin < 100 or TIBC sat <20%
- Sideroblastic anemia:
    - Defective heme synthesis in RBC precursors
    - Hepatosplenomegaly, Fe overload syndromes

- Hereditary/X-linked (ALAS2 mutation), idiopathic, MDS-RARS, reversible causes (**alcohol, lead, isoniazid**, chloramphenicol, copper deficiency, hypothermia)
- Increased iron, normal/high ferritin, normal TIBC
- **Ringed sideroblasts** in bone marrow biopsy (iron laden mitochondria), **Pappenheimer bodies** (Fe inclusions)
- Treatment:
  - Treat reversible causes
  - Trial of pyridoxine 25-50mg PO QD
  - Supportive transfusions

Normocytic:

- Inflammatory anemia- see above
- Sideroblastic anemia- see above
- Pure red cell aplasia:
  - Destructive Ab's or lymphocytes → ineffective erythropoiesis
  - Associated with **thymoma, CLL, parvovirus**
  - Lack of erythroid precursors on bone marrow biopsy
  - Treatment:
    - Thymectomy if thymus enlarged
    - IVIG if parvovirus
    - Immunosuppression for CLL
    - Supportive therapy with PRBCs
- Pancytopenia:
  - Aplastic anemia, hypoplastic myelodysplastic syndrome, myelodysplastic syndrome, aleukemic leukemia, paroxysmal nocturnal hemoglobinuria (PNH), severe megaloblastic anemia, myelofibrosis, metastatic solid tumors, granulomas, hypersplenism, sepsis, alcohol, toxins
  - Fatigue, recurrent infections (neutropenia)
- Aplastic anemia:
  - Stem cell failure
  - Pancytopenia with decreased reticulocytes, bone marrow biopsy with cytogenetics
  - Idiopathic (1/2-1/3), radiation, chemo, chemicals, chloramphenicol, NSAIDs, sulfonamides, drugs, gold, carbamazepine, antithyroid, HHV-6, HIV, EBV, **parvo B19 especially if have sickle cell anemia**, post-hepatitis, SLE, graft vs host disease, thymoma, post hematopoietic stem cell transplant, PNH, Fanconis anemia, shortened telomeres (telomerase mutations)
  - Treatment:
    - Allogenic hematopoietic stem cell transplant for younger patients
    - Cyclosporine/tacrolimus
    - Antithyroid globulin
    - TPO mimetics (eltromopag 50-150mg PO QD) for refractory
    - Supportive transfusions
- Paroxysmal nocturnal hemoglobinuria (PNH):
  - Acquired clonal stem cell disorder → inactivating somatic mutations of PIG-A gene → **deficiency of GPI-anchor for CD55/99 (inhibitors of complement)** → complement mediated RBC lysis with platelet aggregation and subsequent hypercoagulable state

- Intravascular hemolytic anemia with **hypercoagulability** (venous>arterial, especially intra-abdominal (hepatic veins) and cerebral), deficient hematopoiesis, evolution to AML
- During night, retain more CO_2, becomes more acidic, leads to increased complement and increased destruction of RBCs, **urinate red in the morning**
- Use **flow cytometry to show decreased CD55/99**
- Treatment:
  - Folate 3mg/day
  - Eculizumab 900mg IV Q 2 weeks
  - Antithymocyte globulin/cyclosporine A may be needed

Macrocytic:

- Megaloblastic anemia:
  - Impaired DNA synthesis → cytoplasm matures before nucleus → ineffective erythropoiesis and macrocytosis due to folate/B12/MDS
  - Check folate, B12, LDH, and indirect bilirubin
  - Peripheral smear shows **neutrophil hypersegmentation** and **macro-ovalcytes**
- Folate deficiency:
  - Found in vegetables, stores last 2-3 months
  - Malnutrition (alcoholics), decreased absorption (Celiacs), methotrexate, pyrimethamine, trimethoprim
  - Decreased folate, decreased RBC folate, increased homocysteine, **normal methylmalonic acid**
  - Treatment:
    - **Critical to rule out B12 deficiency first**
    - Folate 1-5mg PO QD X 1-4 months
- B12 deficiency:
  - Found in animal foods, 2-3 years of storage
  - **Binds to intrinsic factor from parietal cells, absorbed in the terminal ileum**
  - Malnutrition (vegans, alcoholics), pernicious anemia, decreased absorption (gastrectomy, Crohns, celiacs), *diphyllobothrium latum*
  - **Neurologic changes (subacute combined degeneration),** affects peripheral nerves
  - Posterior/lateral columns affected → numbness, paresthesias, decreased vibratory sensation and positional sense, ataxia, dementia
  - Decreased B12, increased homocysteine, **increased methylmalonic acid**, anti-IF, Schillings test
  - Treatment:
    - B12 1mg IM QD X 7 days, then Q week X 4-8 weeks, then Q month for life

Hemolytic anemias:

- Glucose-6-phosphate dehydrogenase deficiency:
  - X-linked recessive mutation making **RBCs susceptible to oxidative stress**
  - African American males or Mediterranean
  - Drugs (sulfonamides, dapsone, primaquine, doxorubicin, methylene blue), infections, DKA, fava-beans

- o **Heinz bodies** (oxidized Hgb), **bite cells**, decreased G6PD levels
    - G6PD levels may be normal during acute attack, not a good test to order
- o Treatment:
    - Prevention of triggers and avoidance of susceptible meds
    - If severe anemia → transfuse
    - Regular folate supplements
- Sickle cell anemia:
    - o Recessive beta-globulin mutation, decreased O2 causes Hgb to polymerize → RBC sickles → decreased RBC deformability → **hemolysis and microvascular occlusion**
    - o Anemia → chronic hemolysis ± parvo B19 or splenic sequestration crisis
    - o Vaso-occlusion and infarction:
        - **Painful crises, acute chest syndrome**, CVA, dactylitis, renal papillary necrosis, **aseptic necrosis**, priapism
    - o Infection:
        - Splenic infarction leads to **susceptibility to infections from encapsulated organisms** (Strep pneumoniae, H. influenza, Neisseria meningitidis, klebsiella, salmonella typhi, cryptococcus, pseudomonas)
        - Infarcted bone → osteomyelitis (salmonella and staph)
    - o **Sickled RBCs, Howell Jolly bodies, abnormal Hgb electrophoresis**
    - o Treatment:
        - Hydroxyurea 15-35 mg/kg PO QD (increases HgbF)
        - Folate supplements
        - Vaccinations for pneumonia, meningococcus, H. influenza, Hep B
        - Hydration
        - Oxygen and analgesia for acute pain syndrome
        - Exchange transfusions for strokes
        - Penicillin for children
- Hereditary spherocytosis:
    - o Defect in cytoskeletal RBC membrane → **membrane loss, mutations in Ankyrin and alpha/beta spectrins**
    - o Northern European, family history in 75%
    - o Anemia, jaundice, **splenomegaly, pigmented gallstones**
    - o **Spherocytes, + osmotic fragility test, decreased eosin-5-maleimide test**
    - o **Increased MCHC**
    - o Treatment:
        - Folate
        - Transfusions
        - Splenectomy for moderate-severe
- Autoimmune hemolytic anemia (AIHA):
    - o Acquired, **Ab-mediated RBC destruction**
    - o Warm AIHA:
        - **IgG Ab's opsonize RBCs at body temperature** → removed by spleen
        - Idiopathic, **CLL**, non-hodgkins lymphoma, SLE, drugs
    - o Cold AIHA:

- **IgM** Ab binds to RBCs at temperatures < 37C → complement fixation → intravascular hemolysis and acrocyanosis on exposure to cold
- Idiopathic, Waldenstorms macroglobulinemia, **mycoplasma pneumoniae infection, mononucleosis**
  - Diagnosis:
    - Spherocytes, + **Coombs**, cold agglutinin titer, splenomegaly
  - Treatment:
    - Treat underlying disease
    - Warm → corticosteroids $\pm$ splenectomy, IVIG, rituximab
    - Cold → avoid cold, steroids are NOT effective, rituximab
- Drug-induced hemolytic anemia:
  - Acquired, Ab mediated RBC destruction precipitated by a medication
  - Antibiotics- cephalosporins, sulfonamides, rifampin, ribavirin
  - Cardiovascular- **methyldopa**, procainamide, quinidine, thiazides
  - TCAs, phenothiazines, NSAIDs, sulfonylureas, methotrexate, 5-FU, rasbiscurase
  - Diagnosis- **Coomb's negative, increased LDH**
  - Treatment- remove medication
- Microangiopathic hemolytic anemia (MAHA):
  - Intra-arteriolar fibrin damages RBCs → acquired intravascular hemolysis
  - **HUS, TTP, DIC**, malignancy, malignant HTN, **eclampsia/HELLP syndrome, mechanical heart valves,** Sclerodermal renal crisis
  - Diagnosis:
    - **Schistocytes** $\pm$ thrombocytopenia $\pm$ abnormalities in specific diseases (ie increased PT in DIC, increased Cr in HUS, increased LFTs in HELLP)
  - Treatment:
    - Treat underlying disease
    - Emergent plasma exchange for TTP

Transfusion:

- **Goals of blood transfusion:**
  - Increase oxygen delivery to tissues
  - Relieve symptomatic anemia
- **Basic principles:**
  - Decision should NOT be based on hemoglobin value, think of whole clinical picture
  - 1 unit of PRBC increases Hgb by 1
  - American Association of Blood Banks (AABB) guidelines should be used in guiding decision when to transfuse
- **Current AABB guidelines:**
  - Hgb < 6 → transfuse recommended
  - Hgb 6-7 → transfusion likely recommended
  - Hgb 7-8 → restrictive transfusion strategy for stable patients (strong recommendation)

- Consider transfusion only if post-op or symptomatic (chest pain or history of CAD, orthostatic hypotension or tachycardia unresponsive to fluid resuscitation, or CHF)
    - **TRICC trial (1999, NEJM)-** In critically ill patients, restrictive transfusion (Hgb >7) is associated with better survival compared to liberal strategy (Hgb >10)
- **When NOT to transfuse:**
    - Hgb 8-10 → usually NOT indicated
        - Exceptions- ACS with active ischemia, symptomatic anemia, active bleeding, critically ill septic shock with ScVO2 < 70
    - Hgb > 10 → transfusion NOT indicated
- **Risks of blood transfusion:**
    - Transfusion of transmitted pathogens (HIV, HBV, HCV, CMV, bacteria, parasites)
    - Allergic and immunologic reactions
    - Transfusion associated circulatory overload (TACO)
    - Transfusion related acute lung injury (TRALI)
    - Electrolyte abnormalities, hyperkalemia, citrate toxicity (metabolic alkalosis or ionized hypocalcemia)

Risk Factors:

- Poor diet
- Alcoholism
- Drugs
- Infections
- Cancer

Complications:

- Severe fatigue
- High output cardiac failure
- Arrhythmias
- Death

Admission Orders:

- Admit to floor
- Diagnosis anemia
- Condition stable-guarded
- Vital signs routine
- Allergies
- Activity ad lib
- Nursing call for rapidly dropping Hgb/Hct or Hgb <7, HR >110, systolic BP <90
- Diet regular
- Fluids none or PRBCs, fluids per volume assessment
- Meds:
    - Depends on cause
    - Folate 1-5mg PO QD

- B12 1mg IM QD X 7 days
            - Ferrous sulfate 325 PO TID
            - Transfusion as needed
    - Labs/diagnostics:
        - CBC with diff
        - BMP
        - Reticulocyte count
        - RDW
        - Iron studies
            - Fe, TIBC, TIBC sat %, Ferritin
        - Peripheral blood smear
        - B12/folate
        - LDH
        - Haptoglobin
        - Possible bone marrow aspirate/biopsy

Additional Notes:

- Important clinical trials:
    - **TRICC trial (1999, NEJM)-** In critically ill patients, restrictive transfusion (Hgb >7) is associated with better survival compared to liberal strategy (Hgb >10)

Thrombocytopenia

Definitions:

Thrombocytopenia- platelet count <150,000 due to either 1) decreased bone marrow production 2) sequestration of platelets in spleen, or 3) increased platelet destruction

History:

Thrombocytopenia depending on the cause can be asymptomatic, to overt bleeding with organ dysfunction. It can either be suspected based on physical exam findings, from the past medical history if a patient has a disease that makes the person susceptible to thrombocytopenia, or found on laboratory workup. It's important to ask about history of bleeding, family history, recent illnesses, and a thorough medication review.

CC:

HPI:

- COLIDDERRS
- Bleeding?
    - *Where?*
    - *How much?*
- Hx of bleeding?
    - *Describe what it has been like?*
    - *Was it investigated?*
- Recent illness?
    - *ITP can be caused by viral infections, HUS by bacteria*
- Diarrhea?
    - *Symptom of HUS or TTP possibly*
- F/c?
    - *Infectious source can be a cause of thrombocytopenia*
- Heparin treatment in last 5-14 days?
    - *Heparin induced thrombocytopenia*
- Bruising?
    - *Any trauma that caused it?*
- Altered mental status?
    - *Symptom of TTP*
- Neurological symptoms?
    - *Symptom of TTP*

ROS:

PMH:

- Hx of Thrombocytopenia?
    - *What was done for it?*
    - *Was there a diagnosis?*
- Hx of Anemia?
    - *What was done for it?*

- o *Was there a diagnosis?*
- Hx of Renal failure?
    - o *TTP and HUS can cause renal failure*
- Hx of Cirrhosis?
    - o *Common cause of thrombocytopenia*
- Hx of SLE?
    - o *Can cause thrombocytopenia*
- Hx of HIV?
    - o *Common cause of thrombocytopenia*
- Recent illnesses
    - o *Mononucleosis, HUS, ITP, etc.*
- Hx of CLL?
    - o *Can cause thrombocytopenia*

Surgical H:

Social H:

- Alcohol, smoking, recreational drugs, job, living situation, sexual history

Family H:

- Hx of thrombocytopenia, anemia?
    - o *Anything diagnosed?*
    - o *Genetic?*

Allergies:

Medications:

- Heparin recently?
- Chemotherapy medications?
- Quinine or sulfonamides?

Physical Examination:

The physical exam should look for findings that are either sequelae of thrombocytopenia, or findings that can be associated with diseases causing thrombocytopenia.

- Vital signs
- Petechiae?
    - o Common sign of thrombocytopenia
- Altered mental status?
    - o HUS and TTP
- Enlarged spleen?
    - o Cirrhosis, ITP, TTP, CLL etc have enlarged spleen due to splenic sequestration
- Liver exam
    - o Cirrhosis liver will be small
- Wet purpura?
    - o ITP, TTP
- Oral mucosa blisters?

- - HIV, infections, etc.
- Focal neurological symptoms?
  - TTP
- Retinal hemorrhages?
  - Poor prognostic sign in ITP

Differential Diagnosis:

- See etiology

Labs:

- CBC with diff
  - Look for plt count, anemia, leukocytosis/leukopenia
- Peripheral smear
  - Increased destruction shows schistocytes
  - Decreased production shows blasts
- Platelet count in non-EDTA tubes to rule out pseuodothrombocytopenia
- If anemic:
  - Reticulocyte count
  - LDH
  - Haptoglobin
  - Indirect bilirubin
- If hemolytic anemia:
  - PT, PTT
  - Fibrinogen
    - Decreased in DIC
  - D-dimer
    - Elevated in DIC
  - Coombs test
    - ITP will be positive
  - ANA
    - Screen for SLE
- HIV test
- Hep C RNA
  - Cause of cirrhosis chronically
- Bone marrow biopsy for unexplained thrombocytopenia, especially if splenomegaly is present

Imaging:

- Possibly liver US if suspecting cirrhosis, and spleen US for sequestration

Algorithm for Thrombocytopenia Evaluation:

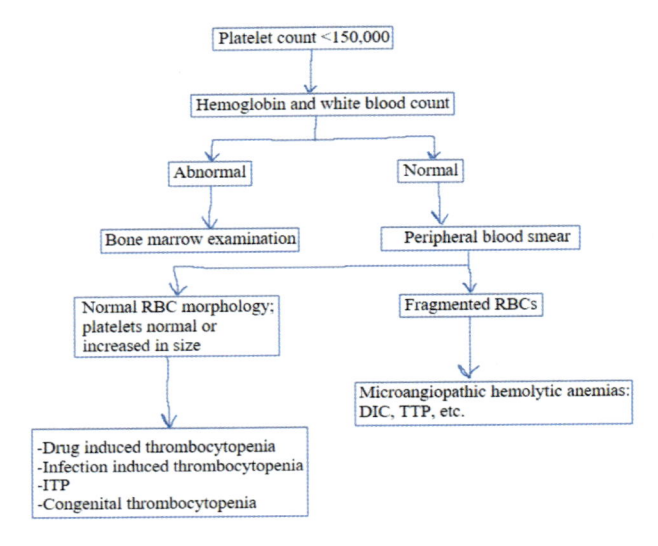

```
Platelet count <150,000
        │
        ▼
Hemoglobin and white blood count
   │              │
Abnormal        Normal
   │              │
   ▼              ▼
Bone marrow    Peripheral blood smear
examination       │         │
   │              ▼         ▼
   │         Normal RBC morphology;   Fragmented RBCs
   │         platelets normal or          │
   │         increased in size            ▼
   │              │              Microangiopathic hemolytic anemias:
   │              │              DIC, TTP, etc.
   ▼              ▼
-Drug induced thrombocytopenia
-Infection induced thrombocytopenia
-ITP
-Congenital thrombocytopenia
```

Etiologies/Pathogenesis/Symptoms/Diagnosis/Treatment:

- Infection induced thrombocytopenia:
    - Can have DIC with this
    - Most common cause is viral
    - Can be gram negative rods, **infectious mononucleosis, early HIV**
    - Might have to do bone marrow biopsy
    - Treatment:
        - Treat underlying disorder, usually self-limited
- Drug-induced thrombocytopenia:
    - Chemotherapy drugs, herbal drugs, over the counter drugs
    - Quinine and sulfonamides cause drug dependent antibodies that react with platelet surface antigens
        - Takes 21 days to show, and resolves after 7 days of stopping the drug
    - Treatment:
        - Stop the medication
- Heparin induced thrombocytopenia (HIT):
    - Usually not severe thrombocytopenia (rarely <20,000)
    - **NOT** associated with bleeding
    - **Causes a hypercoagulable state** (arterial>venous)
    - **Anti-heparin/PF4 antibody complex activates platelets**
    - Can occur with low molecular weight heparin or unfractionated heparin, usually **5-14 days after starting the medication**
    - Diagnosis:
        - Anti-hep/PF4 antibody assay with ELISA
        - Serotonin release assay
    - Treatment:
        - Early recognition is key

- **Discontinue heparin**
- Replace with direct thrombin inhibitor **argatroban** 2 mcg/kg/min IV, or lepirudin or fondaparinux
- If get thrombosis, do anticoagulation for 3-6 months
- Start warfarin after resolution of thrombocytopenia for 3-6 months
  - Investigate for lower/upper extremity DVTs with Doppler US
  - If on warfarin, give vitamin K
  - Platelet transfusions do NOT help
- Immune thrombocytopenic purpura (ITP):
  - Acquired thrombocytopenia with **immune mediated destruction of platelets and inhibition of platelet release from megakaryocytes**
  - Children- post infection and self-limited
  - Adults- more chronic, can be from underlying disorder (SLE, HIV, Hep C, H. pylori), women>males
  - **Insidious onset of mucocutaneous bleeding**
  - **Very low platelet count**
  - Normal blood cells and peripheral smear
  - Wet purpura and retinal hemorrhages may herald life threatening bleeding is present
  - Diagnosis
    - Antibody test NOT good
    - Diagnosis of exclusion
    - Tests for HIV, Hep C, SLE, Ig levels, H. pylori antibodies, and Coomb's test
    - Bone marrow exam reserved for signs/labs not explained by ITP or those not responding to therapy
  - Treatment:
    - With no bleeding, platelet count <5,000, and no signs of impending bleeding, treat outpatient with prednisone 1mg/kg or WinRho SDF 50-75 µg/kg
    - With severe ITP and bleeding, admit, and use high dose glucocorticoids (methylprednisolone) and IVIG, possibly with rituximab
    - Splenectomy for patients who relapse after glucocorticoids are tapered, then vaccinate for S. pneumoniae, meningococcal, and H. influenza
    - Eltrombopag or romiplostim for patients who relapse after splenectomy
    - For bleeding, use aminocaproic acid, methylprednisolone, IVIG
    - **Platelet transfusions do NOT help**
- Thrombotic thrombocytopenic purpura (TTP), Hemolytic uremic syndrome (HUS), and DIC:
  - **Schistocytes**, lab evidence of hemolysis (**increased LDH, decreased haptoglobin, increased indirect bilirubin**), microvascular thrombosis
  - DIC:
    - **All lab hematologic lab values abnormal** (increased PTT, increased PT, decreased fibrinogen, etc.)
    - **Bleeding/oozing from everywhere**
    - **Schistocytes**

- If the **patient has cirrhosis, check factor VIII level** (will be increased in cirrhotic patients, normal in DIC patients)
- Fix underlying disease, and give blood products
  - If decreased fibrinogen → cryoprecipitate (goal >100)
  - If increased INR → FFP
  - If decreased platelets → platelets (goal >50)
  - If decreased Hgb → PRBCs

- TTP:
  - **Pentad (FAT RN):**
    - Fever
    - Anemia (microangiopathic hemolytic anemia)
    - Thrombocytopenia
    - Renal failure
    - Neurologic symptoms
  - **Deficiency of ADAMTS13**, which normally cleaves Von Willebrand factor units
    - This causes VWF to be very large as the units cannot be cleaved
    - These long VWF units will fragment RBCs, causing **schistocytes**, as well as causing platelet adhesion and aggregation and **microvascular thrombosis**
  - Can do lab tests for ADAMTS13 activity
  - Normal PT/PTT unlike DIC, normal fibrinogen, normal split products
  - Idiopathic TTP- women, HIV, pregnancy, ticlopidine use, clopidogrel use
  - Treatment of TTP:
    - Need labs to rule out DIC
    - **Plasmapheresis**
    - **Glucocorticoids** as an adjunct
    - **Caplacizumab** has been shown to treat acquired TTP more rapidly than conventional treatment (NEJM Vol. 374m No. 6, Pg. 511) by rapidly blocking Von Willebrand factor mediated platelet aggregation
    - If refractory, rituximab, vincristine, cyclophosphamide, and splenectomy
    - **Platelet transfusions do NOT help**

- HUS:
  - Has more renal failure than TTP and usually no neurological symptoms
  - **Bloody diarrhea, usually from E. coli O157:H7**
  - Shiga toxin activates endothelium leading to activation of VWF, and causing platelet aggregation and thrombocytopenia
  - Treatment:
    - Supportive therapy
    - Dialysis is needed in ~40% of patients
    - Possible eclizumab therapy

- Inherited thrombocytopenia:

- Rare
  - Nonmuscle myosin heavy chain MYH9 gene, **Wiskott-Aldrich syndrome, Bernard soulier disease**

Risk Factors:

- Infections with HIV, Hep C
- Heparin use
- SLE

Complications:

- Bleeding
- Death

Additional Notes:

-

Transient Ischemic Attacks and Ischemic Stroke

Definitions:

Transient ischemic attack- episodes of stroke symptoms lasting <24 hours, with most lasting <1 hour, with normal brain imaging caused by cerebral ischemia

Ischemic stroke- sudden loss of blood circulation to an area of the brain from thrombotic or embolic occlusion of a cerebral artery, resulting in a corresponding loss of neurologic function

TIA

History and physical- see ischemic stroke

Differential diagnosis- ischemic/hemorrhagic stroke, seizure, migraine, hypoglycemia, amyloid spells, transposition of great arteries, anxiety, syncope, Meniere's disease

Risk of recurrence:

- **ABCD^2 Score- the 3 month rate of stroke after a TIA**
    - **A**ge $\geq$ 60 (1)
    - Systolic **B**P >140 or diastolic BP >90 (1)
    - **C**linical features of TIA:
        - Unilateral weakness (2)
        - Speech disturbance without weakness (1)
    - **D**uration:
        - Lasting >60 minutes (2)
        - Lasting 10-59 minutes (1)
    - **D**iabetes (1)
    - **Admit the patient if:**
        - Score is $\geq$ 3
        - Score is 0-2 and uncertain if diagnostic workup can be done as an outpatient
        - Score is 0-2 and other evidence that the event was caused by focal ischemia
- Rates of recurrence based on score:
    - 0- 0%
    - 1- 2%
    - 2- 3%
    - 3- 3%
    - 4- 8%
    - 5- 12%
    - 6- 17%
    - 7- 22%

Treatment- See ischemic stroke treatment below

Ischemic Stroke

History:

When someone comes in to the ED with a suspected stroke, it is important to know the timeframe when symptoms began and/or lasted, what symptoms they have, and any risk factors they might have for a stroke. The timeframe is important because that can change the acute treatment course. It's also important to try and differentiate stroke symptoms with seizure symptoms.

CC:

HPI:

- COLIDDERRS
    - *Focal neurologic deficit, acute HTN, diabetes, obese, smoker, vascular disease (thrombotic), A-fib with valvular disease (embolic)*
    - *Think of **FAST** → facial droop, arm drift, slurred speech, time and transport*
- Specific symptoms
- Onset of symptoms
    - *This is important to whether tPA can be used (can do if ≤ 4.5 hours since start of symptoms, better if before 3 hours)*
- Sensory loss?
    - *Where?*
    - *For how long?*
- Motor loss? Unilateral?
    - *Where*
- Vision changes?
    - *Symptom of a stroke*
- Gait changes?
    - *Motor weakness from stoke or cerebellar dysfunction*
- Slurred speech?
    - *Common symptom of stroke*
- Headache?
    - *Can be a sign of hypertension and possible hemorrhagic stroke too*
- Seizure like activity?
    - *Possibly could be a seizure*
- Tongue biting?
    - *Can be a sign of seizure*
- Urinary incontinence?
    - *Can be a sign of stroke, seizure, or any neurological disease*

ROS:

PMH:

- Hx of TIA/stroke?
    - *What was done?*
    - *Residual deficits?*
- Hx of Atrial fibrillation?

- o *Causes ~20% of ischemic strokes*
- Hx of Diabetes?
  - o *Risk factor for ischemic stroke*
- Hx of Dyslipidemia?
  - o *Risk factor for ischemic stroke*
- Hx of HTN?
  - o *Biggest risk factor for ischemic stroke*
- Hx of Seizures?
  - o *May mimic a stroke*
- Hx of Neurological diseases?
  - o *Can cause symptoms of stroke or bowel incontinence too*

Surgical H:

Social H:

- Alcohol, **smoking**, recreational drugs, job, living situation, sexual history

Family H:

Allergies:

Medications:

- Birth control?
  - o *Risk to cause clots*
- Hormone replacement therapy (estrogen)?
  - o *Risk to cause clots*

Physical Examination:

It's important to do a quick physical exam to assess for focal neurological symptoms. Vital signs are important as elevated blood pressure may change the course of management.

- Vital signs
  - o Look for hypertension that needs to be treated and also contraindicates the use of tPA (systolic BP > 185)
- Arrhythmias?
  - o A-fib
- Murmurs?
  - o Can predispose to clots forming
- Carotid/subclavian bruits?
  - o Atherosclerotic plaques that can embolize to the brain
- Full neuro exam
  - o CN's, strength, reflexes, sensory, etc.

Differential Diagnosis:

- TIA
  - o *Stroke symptoms lasting <24 hours*
- Ischemic stroke
- Intracranial hemorrhage

- o   *Focal neurological deficit with the worst headache of their life*
- Subdural hematoma
  - o   *Older person with minimal trauma who has headache and classic findings on CT (crescenteric shaped)*
- Epidural hematoma
  - o   *Person with head trauma who loses consciousness, regains consciousness, and then quickly decompensates with classic findings on CT (lens shaped)*
- Seizure (Todd's paralysis)
  - o   *Person who has a seizure and has a post-ictal hemi paralysis that may mimic an acute stroke*
- Brain tumor
  - o   *Headaches, nausea, vision changes, possible other cancer that has not metastasized, change in personality*
- Migraine
  - o   *No risk factors for stroke, aura, n/v, light and sound intolerance, no CT findings*
- Vertigo
  - o   *Dizziness, room can be spinning, etc.*
- Hypoglycemia
  - o   *Can cause LOC, seizure like activity, sensory abnormalities, usually in a diabetic who takes insulin*
- Guillain Barre syndrome
  - o   *2-4 weeks after a respiratory or GI illness, who complains of finger tingling, proximal muscle weakness of lower extremities, which then starts to affect arms, trunk, CNs, and muscles of respiration*
- Multiple sclerosis
  - o   *Younger female who has multiple neurologic complaints that are not pinpoint, vision changes, and these happen intermittently over time*
- Aortic dissection
  - o   *Sudden onset of severe chest pain, may be anterior chest pain or radiate to the back depending where the dissection is, tearing or ripping pain, can have neurological symptoms*

Acute Labs:

- CBC
  - o   Look for anemia which could show bleeding, plt count
- CMP
  - o   Look for electrolyte abnormalities, hypoglycemia
- Troponins
  - o   Cardiac ischemia could be occurring
- Toxicology screen
  - o   Loss of conscious could be from drugs
- PT/PTT/INR
  - o   Need to see if can use tPA
- Glucose
  - o   For hypoglycemia

Acute Imaging:

- EKG

- o   For acute ischemia
- Stat non-contrast CT of head to rule out intracranial hemorrhage
  - o   Need to see if can use tPA, may be able to see the ischemic stroke, may see hemorrhage, subdural/epidural hematoma

Workup for Etiology/Modifiable Risk Factors:

- Cardiac- EKG, continuous telemetry, echo (thrombus or vegetation) with bubble study (PFO), holter monitor outpatient if arrhythmia not captured if feel is due to A-fib
- Vessel imaging- carotid US and Doppler
- MRI- better than CT for ischemic stroke
- Labs- lipids, HbA1c, TSH, ESR/CRP, blood cultures if systemic signs and symptoms are present

Algorithm for Stroke/TIA Management:

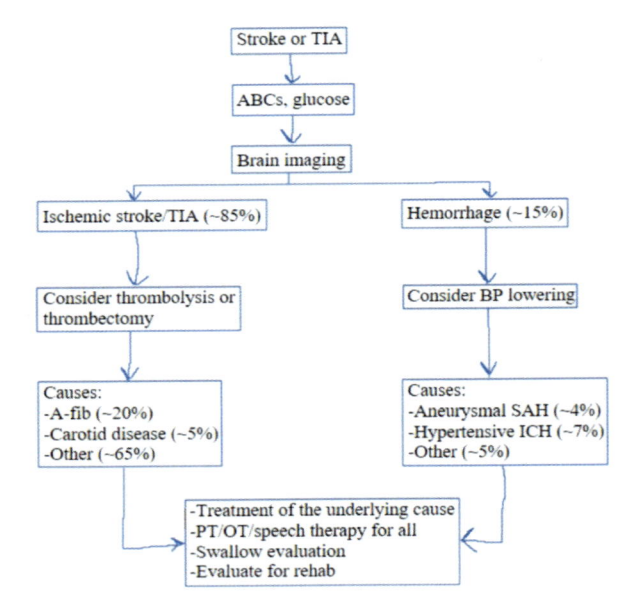

```
Stroke or TIA
    ↓
ABCs, glucose
    ↓
Brain imaging
    ↓
    ├─────────────────────────────┐
    ↓                             ↓
Ischemic stroke/TIA (~85%)    Hemorrhage (~15%)
    ↓                             ↓
Consider thrombolysis or      Consider BP lowering
thrombectomy
    ↓                             ↓
Causes:                       Causes:
-A-fib (~20%)                 -Aneurysmal SAH (~4%)
-Carotid disease (~5%)        -Hypertensive ICH (~7%)
-Other (~65%)                 -Other (~5%)
```

-Treatment of the underlying cause
-PT/OT/speech therapy for all
-Swallow evaluation
-Evaluate for rehab

Treatment of Ischemic Stroke:

Acute Treatment of Ischemic Stroke:

- 1st goal is to **prevent or reverse brain injury, ABCs, treat hypo/hyperglycemia, and non-contrast head CT**
- Treat malignant HTN if present (>185/110)
  - o   Use IV esmolol 1000 mcg/kg X1, then 150mcg/kg/min
- **IV rTpA** 0.9 mg/kg, max 90mg, 10% as a bolus, rest over 60 minute, **indications (all must be present):**

- Clinical diagnosis of stroke
- Onset of signs/symptoms ≤ **4.5 hours** (better if within 3 hours)
- CT with no hemorrhage or edema of >1/3 of the MCA territory
- Consent
- **NINDS trial (1995, NEJM)-** In patients with stroke <u>within 3 hours</u>, tPA administration significantly improved NIHSS scores but did not confer survival benefit
- **ECASS III trial (2008, NEJM)-** IV alteplase improved neurologic outcomes <u>within 4.5 hours</u> of stroke onset among patients with acute ischemic stroke. Despite an increased incidence of intracranial hemorrhage, there was no mortality benefit.

- **Contraindications (absolute) for thrombolytics:**
    - Any prior intracranial hemorrhage
    - Brain tumor/aneurysm/AVM
    - Systolic BP >185
    - Ischemic stroke within 3 months
    - Active bleeding except menses
    - Suspected aortic dissection
- Permissive hypertension as tolerable (~140-180 SBP)
- Endovascular revascularization:
    - Thrombolytics directly to the thrombus, can be **up to 6 hours** from onset of signs/symptoms
    - Mechanical thrombolectomy for ineligible or have contraindications to thrombolysis, or thrombolysis failed
- **Aspirin within 48 hours of onset of stroke, consider Plavix in addition:**
    - **IST trial (1997, The Lancet)-** The administration of aspirin within 48 hours of ischemic stroke onset reduces the risk of 14-day recurrence and the combined outcome of nonfatal stroke or death
    - **CHANCE trial (2013, NEJM)-** Among patients with acute TIA or minor ischemic stroke, starting aspirin/clopidogrel within 24h of symptom onset reduces the 90-day stroke incidence without increasing bleeding rates, when compared to aspirin monotherapy
        - Current guidelines still recommend aspirin alone, but may be changing
    - **CHARISMA trial (2006, NEJM)-** Among patients at high risk for cardiovascular events, combination aspirin plus clopidogrel did not significantly reduce the rates of MI, stroke, or death from CV causes. There was increased bleeding with combination therapy.
- Aggrenox (ASA/dipyridamole) if patient had stroke while on aspirin
    - **ESPRIT trial (2006, The Lancet)-** In patients with TIAs or minor ischemic strokes, combination aspirin/dipyridamole was associated with lower rates of vascular mortality, non-fatal stroke, non-fatal MI, and non-fatal major bleeding when compared to aspirin alone
- Statin therapy
    - **SPARCL trial (2006, NEJM)-** In patients with prior stroke/TIA, atorvastatin reduces the risk of recurrent ischemic stroke, but may increase risk of hemorrhagic stroke
- ACEI
    - **HOPE trial (2000, NEJM)-** Ramipril reduces the rate of death, MI, and stroke among patients with multiple CV risk factors and without heart failure
- Water restriction and IV mannitol on $2^{nd}/3^{rd}$ day for edema prevention
- NO anticoagulation with heparin or warfarin, does not help

- Stroke centers and rehab referral, the earlier the better
- Acetaminophen to prevent fever
- SSRI therapy within 5-10 days of stroke onset has been shown to improve motor recovery
    - **FLAME (Stroke) trial (2011, The Lancet Neurology)-** Early administration of fluoxetine (initiated 5-10 days after stroke onset) in addition to conventional physiotherapy improves motor recovery in patients with moderate to severe motor deficits due to ischemic stroke
        - Although, no guidelines have been published reflecting these results
- **Core measures to be done in hospital:**
    - PT evaluation and treatment
    - OT evaluation and treatment
    - ST evaluation for swallow study (keep NPO until done)
    - Anti-platelet by day 2
    - CT or MRI of the brain
    - Carotid ultrasound and echo
    - Statin
    - ACEI

Primary/Secondary Prevention of Stroke/TIA:

- BP control:
    - Best is <140/90
    - Thiazides and ACEIs have the best support (see above HOPE trial for ACEI)
    - **SPS3-BP trial (2013, The Lancet)-** Among patients with a recent lacunar stroke (here, small subcortical stroke or S3), lower-target BP control (target SBP <130) does not reduce incident of stroke when compared to higher-target BP control (target 140-150). However, there was a non-significant trend towards benefit (P=0.08).
- High dose statins- atorvastatin 40-80mg PO QHS
- Smoking cessation
- Aspirin 81mg PO QD for life, OR
- Clopidogrel QD for life
    - Has been shown to be superior to aspirin, but increases the risk of bleeding
- Can add dipyridamole if stroke occurred while on aspirin
- Atrial fibrillation treatment:
    - Xarelto, eliquis, pradaxa, savayasa (see clinical trials in AF section)
    - Warfarin tailored for INR 2-3
- Carotid atherosclerosis treatment:
    - Endarterectomy- within 2 weeks for someone with stenosis 70-99% with symptoms
    - Endovascular stent- for patients not suitable for endarterectomy
- Diabetes treatment
    - Goal A1c < 7.0

Etiology:

- Cardioembolic stroke:
    - ~20% of ischemic strokes

- Most often affects the middle cerebral artery
- Atrial fibrillation, MI, prosthetic valves, right heart disease, paradoxical embolus
- Carotid atherosclerosis:
  - Thrombosis
  - Lacunar infarction
- Other causes:
  - Hypercoagulable disorders, venous sinus thrombosis, fibromuscular dysplasia, vasculitis, sickle cell disease, aortic dissection

Risk Factors:

- Older age
- **Hypertension** (most important risk factor)
- Diabetes
- Smoking
- Low HDL
- High LDL
- Prior TIA/stroke
- Atrial fibrillation
- Birth control involving estrogen

Pathogenesis:

- Decreased blood flow to brain, zero blood flow for 4-10 minutes causes death of brain tissue
- Necrotic pathway and apoptotic pathway activated
- Ischemia → necrosis → no glucose or oxygen to brain cells → failure of mitochondria to produce ATP → membrane ion pumps stop → intracellular calcium is increased → glutamate is released → more calcium influx → apoptosis
- Free radicals are produced which destroy the cellular membranes and injure the mitochondrial membranes causing apoptosis

Complications:

- Permanent paralysis or loss of muscle movement
- Difficulty talking or swallowing (aspiration risk)
- Memory loss
- Emotional problems (depression)
- Chronic pain
- Changes in behavior and self-care ability

Admission Orders:

- Admit to floor/ICU
- Diagnosis acute ischemic stroke/TIA
- Condition guarded
- Vital signs Q4h, neuro checks Q2h for 1st 24h then Q4h, call for temp >38C, systolic BP >200 or <120, HR >100
- Allergies

- Activity bedrest until initial physical therapy assessment is performed, then mobilize ASAP as guided by PT, strict fall precautions
- Nursing supplemental O2 to maintain >93%, check capillary blood glucose Q6h
- Diet NPO until swallow evaluation is done, then heart healthy if cleared
- Fluids
- Meds:
    - Aspirin 325mg PO QD within 48 hours
    - Acetaminophen 650mg Q6h for 48h to prevent fever
    - tPa if within 4.5 hours (preferably 3 hours)
- Labs/diagnostics:
    - Non-contrast CT of head
    - CBC with platelets
    - PT/PTT/INR
    - CMP
    - EKG
    - Carotid duplex and echo next day

Discharge Information:

- Must be neurologically stable
- Must be able to eat or have a feeding tube
- PT/OT determine what facility to go to patient goes to
- Have a safe home environment if going home
- Speech pathology evaluation
- Aspirin and/or clopidogrel or aggrenox
- High dose statin
- ACEI
- Consider SSRI
- Follow up in 2 weeks with PCP and neurology

Additional Notes:

- Important clinical trials:
    - **IST trial (1997, The Lancet)-** The administration of aspirin within 48 hours of ischemic stroke onset reduces the risk of 14-day recurrence and the combined outcome of nonfatal stroke or death
    - **CHANCE trial (2013, NEJM)-** Among patients with acute TIA or minor ischemic stroke, starting aspirin/clopidogrel within 24h of symptom onset reduces the 90-day stroke incidence without increasing bleeding rates, when compared to aspirin monotherapy
        - Current guidelines still recommend aspirin alone, but may be changing
    - **CHARISMA trial (2006, NEJM)-** Among patients at high risk for cardiovascular events, combination aspirin plus clopidogrel did not significantly reduce the rates of MI, stroke, or death from CV causes. There was increased bleeding with combination therapy.
    - **NINDS trial (1995, NEJM)-** In patients with stroke within 3 hours, tPA administration significantly improved NIHSS scores but did not confer survival benefit
    - **ECASS III trial (2008, NEJM)-** IV alteplase improved neurologic outcomes within 4.5 hours of stroke onset among patients with acute

ischemic stroke. Despite an increased incidence of intracranial hemorrhage, there was no mortality benefit.
- **ESPRIT trial (2006, The Lancet)-** In patients with TIAs or minor ischemic strokes, combination aspirin/dipyridamole was associated with lower rates of vascular mortality, non-fatal stroke, non-fatal MI, and non-fatal major bleeding when compared to aspirin alone
- **SPARCL trial (2006, NEJM)-** In patients with prior stroke/TIA, atorvastatin reduces the risk of recurrent ischemic stroke, but may increase risk of hemorrhagic stroke
- **HOPE trial (2000, NEJM)-** Ramipril reduces the rate of death, MI, and stroke among patients with multiple CV risk factors and without heart failure
- **FLAME (Stroke) trial (2011, The Lancet Neurology)-** Early administration of fluoxetine (initiated 5-10 days after stroke onset) in addition to conventional physiotherapy improves motor recovery in patients with moderate to severe motor deficits due to ischemic stroke
    - Although, no guidelines have been published reflecting these results
- **SPS3-BP trial (2013, The Lancet)-** Among patients with a recent lacunar stroke (here, small subcortical stroke or S3), lower-target BP control (target SBP <130) does not reduce incident of stroke when compared to higher-target BP control (target 140-150). However, there was a non-significant trend towards benefit (P=0.08).

Acute Confusion/Delirium

Definitions:

Confusion- a mental and behavioral state of reduced comprehension, coherence, and capacity to reason

Delirium- a relatively acute decline in cognition that fluctuates over hours-days

History:

The history is the most important piece to a patient who is presenting with acute confusion or delirium. It is invaluable as well to have a collateral source available to discuss the patients' current state and how they are at their baseline. There are three very important details to know in this patient population; **1) patients baseline cognitive function, 2) time course of present illness**, and **3) current medications** (new meds, dose, recent changes, etc.).

CC:

HPI:

- COLIDDERRS
- **What is the patients' baseline cognitive function?**
    - *Need to know how different the patients current state is compared to baseline, as someone with dementia may be at their baseline already*
- **Time course of present illness**
    - *Acute is more likely to be delirium whereas ongoing over a period of time is more likely to be dementia*
- Review outpatient records
    - *Very important to get their PMHx*
- Any recent illness?
    - *Infection can be a cause of acute delirium*
- Illicit drug use?
    - *Drugs can be a cause of psychosis, delirium, etc.*
- Toxin exposures?
    - *Alcohol, CO, ethylene glycol, inhalants, pesticides, etc.*
- Head trauma?
    - *Subdural hematoma, epidural hematoma, etc.*
- Hydration status
    - *Dehydration can cause delirium, electrolyte abnormalities can occur with dehydration or fluid overload (Na and Ca abnormalities)*

ROS:

PMH:

- **Very important to get the full past medical history**
- Hx of Organ failure?
    - *Cirrhosis can cause hepatic encephalopathy*

- CKD can cause uremia
- Hx of Alcoholism?
  - Acute alcohol toxicity or Wernicke Korsakoff syndrome
- Hx of CHF?
  - Can cause altered mental status in acute decompensation, can cause kidney failure overtime as well as cirrhosis
- Hx of Depression?
  - Can lead to drug abuse, possible drug overdose
- Hx of Malignancy?
  - Mets to the brain can cause encephalopathy and personality changes

Surgical H:

Social H:

- **Alcohol**, smoking, **recreational drugs**, job, living situation, sexual history

Family H:

Allergies:

Medications:

- **Extremely important to review all medications and their doses**
- Any recent medication changes?
- Anticholinergics, narcotics, benzodiazepines are common meds that can cause delirium, they should also for the most part be avoided in elderly patients

Physical Examination:

Vital signs are the most important piece of the physical exam in a patient with confusion/delirium. A full physical exam should be done to look for any clues that may be causing the patients current state.

- Vital signs
  - Look for fever, hypotension, hypertension, tachycardia
- Respiratory exam
  - Consolidation, rales, crackles
- Cardiac exam
- Stiff neck?
  - Brudzinski and Kernigs for meningitis
- Fluid status
- Skin
  - Jaundice, cyanosis, needle tracks
- Full neuro and mental status exam
  - Digit span test for attention deficits (repeat #'s, adding one # each time, normal person can repeat 5-7 numbers)
  - Spell world backwards
  - GCS, MMSE, confusion assessment method

Differential Diagnosis:

- See etiology

Labs:

- Usually are guided by the H&P
- **Labs everyone gets:**
    - CBC
        - Look for anemia, leukocytosis
    - CMP
        - Look for electrolyte abnormalities, hypoglycemia, abnormal LFTs, elevated BUN and Cr
    - TSH
        - Hypo/hyperthyroidism can cause delirium
    - Glucose levels
- Others guided by history:
    - Blood cultures
        - If you think an infection is the cause
    - UA with culture
        - If you think UTI is the cause
    - Serum/urine toxicology screen
        - If drugs are thought to be the cause
    - ABG
        - If patient is in any respiratory distress, may need to be intubated
    - Ammonia level
        - Rarely useful, helps to point to a hepatic cause
    - B12
        - If you suspect alcoholism
    - ESR
        - If infection is suspected
    - Autoimmune serologies (ANA, complement, P/C-ANCA)
        - If other sources are not found
    - RPR
        - If syphilis is thought to be the cause
    - HIV antibody
        - If HIV is suspected

Imaging:

- EKG for all
    - In case decreased perfusion to the brain is occurring from decreased cardiac output from myocardial ischemia
- Elderly → CXR
    - Looking for pneumonia
- Head CT, followed by MRI if necessary
    - Looking for any intracranial etiologies
- Possibly neck X-ray
    - If trauma of neck has occurred
- Possibly EEG
    - If seizures are thought to be the cause

Treatment:

- **Treat underlying cause** once found (see etiology)
- Avoid benzodiazepines/antipsychotics
- Can use precedex (dexmedetomidine)
- **Empiric treatment (TONG)**, if necessary:
    - **T**hiamine 100mg IV prior to dextrose
    - **O**xygen
    - **N**aloxone 0.01mg/kg if suspect opiate overdose
    - **G**lucose (Dextrose 50g IV push)
- Further empiric therapy/ancillary therapy:
    - Address sensory/cognitive impairment
    - Increase familiarity of current setting (bring in pictures, things from patients room)
    - Decrease/prevent physical restraints
    - Prevent infections and remove lines/catheters if possible
    - Promote good sleep:
        - Reduce noise and night time interventions
        - Open windows during the day

Etiology:

- **HE STOPS TIPS AEIOU:**
    - **H**TN/**H**epatic
    - **E**lectrolytes
    - **S**troke
    - **T**rauma
    - **O**piates
    - **P**sych
    - **S**eizure
    - **T**emperature
    - **I**nfection
    - **P**orphyria
    - **S**epsis
    - **A**cidosis
    - **E**ndocrine
    - **I**ntoxication
    - **O**xygen
    - **U**remia
- Toxins:
    - Prescription medications:
        - Anticholinergics
        - Narcotics
        - Benzodiazepines
    - Drugs of abuse:
        - Alcohol
            - *Emotional instability, slurred speech, ataxia*
        - Opiates
            - *Euphoria, respiratory and CNS depression, pinpoint pupils*
        - Ecstasy
            - *Euphoria*
        - LSD

- *Visual and auditory perceptual distortions, depersonalization, anxiety, paranoia, flashbacks*
  - GHB
    - *Euphoria, sedation*
  - PCP
    - *Belligerence, impulsiveness, fever, psychosis, nystagmus*
  - Ketamine
    - *Hallucinations*
  - Cocaine
    - *Impaired judgement, pupillary dilation, hallucinations, paranoid*
  - Bath salts
    - *Aggressive*
  - Marijuana
    - *Conjunctival injection, hunger, euphoria, perception of slowed time, slowed reflexes, dry mouth*
- Poisons:
  - Inhalants
  - CO
    - *Headache, fatigue, barbeque exposure or running car*
  - Ethylene glycol
    - *Usually seen ingesting, may be asymptomatic, will develop altered mental status and dyspnea*
  - Pesticides
    - *Initial euphoria with auditory or visual hallucinations, seizures, agitation, lethargy, unconsciousness, n/v, skin rash,*

- Metabolic conditions:
  - Electrolyte disturbances:
    - Hypo/hyperglycemia
    - Hypo/hypernatremia
    - Hypocalcemia/hypercalcemia
    - Hypomagnesia
  - Hypo/hyperthermia
  - Respiratory failure:
    - Hypoxemia
    - Hypercapnia
  - Liver failure and hepatic encephalopathy
  - Renal failure and uremia
  - Cardiac failure
  - Vit B12, thiamine, folate, and niacin deficiency
  - Dehydration
  - Malnutrition
  - Anemia
- Infections:
  - Systemic:
    - UTI
    - Pneumonia

- Skin/soft tissue infections
- Sepsis
  - CNS:
    - Meningitis
    - Encephalitis
    - Brain abscess
- Endocrine conditions:
  - Hypo/hyperthyroidism
  - Hyperparathyroidism
  - Adrenal insufficiency
- Cerebrovascular disorders:
  - Global hypoperfusion states
  - Hypertensive encephalopathy
  - Focal ischemic stroke and hemorrhages
- Autoimmune disorders:
  - Cerebral lupus
  - CNS vasculitis
  - Neurologic paraneoplastic syndromes
- Seizure-related disorders:
  - Non-convulsive status epilepticus
  - Intermittent seizures with prolonged postictal states
- Neoplastic disorders:
  - Diffuse metastases to the brain
  - Gliomatosis cerebri
  - Carcinomatous meningitis
  - CNS lymphoma
- Psychological:
  - Psychosis
  - Fake
- Porphyria
- Hospitalization
- Terminal end of life delirium

Risk Factors:

- Age (>65)
- Low scores on standardized tests of cognition
- Pre-existing hearing/visual impairments
- Baseline immobility
- Malnutrition
- Underlying medical/neurologic illness
- Dementia at baseline
- In hospital risks:
  - Bladder catheterization
  - Physical restraints
  - Sleep/sensory deprivation
  - Addition of 3 or more new medications
  - Cardiopulmonary bypass
  - Inadequate or excessive treatment of pain
  - Some inhaled anesthetics

Pathogenesis:

- Attention deficit which is hallmark has a diffuse localization within the brainstem thalamus, prefrontal cortex, and parietal lobes
- EEG shows symmetric slowing
- **Deficiency of acetylcholine**
- **Increase in dopamine** (visual hallucinations)
- Mechanism not fully understood

Complications:

- General decline in health
- Poor recovery from surgery
- Need for nursing home
- Increased risk of death
- Permanent neurologic sequalae

Additional Notes:

-

Approach to the Acutely Ill Infected Febrile Patient

History:

When you have a patient who is febrile and it is evident that they have an infection, it is important to determine what type of infection so empiric treatment can be implemented.

CC:

HPI:

- COLIDDERRS
- Onset of symptoms?
- Duration?
- Changes since onset?
    - *Tell if they are getting better or worse, if getting better may not need to change much about their treatment*
- Progression?
    - *How has it progressed*
- Asplenic?
    - *Leaves them susceptible to encapsulated organisms (H. influenza type b, strep pneumoniae, N. meningitidis, group B strep, klebsiella, salmonella typhi)*
- Recent illness?
    - *What was it and was it treated?*
- Chemotherapy?
    - *Makes them more susceptible to infections when they are in an immunocompromised state*
- Cuts?
    - *Potential source of cellulitis, osteomyelitis, necrotizing fasciitis, etc.*
- Burns?
    - *Can leave you susceptible to pseudomonas*
- Trauma?
    - *Potential sites for infection*
- Sick contacts?
    - *What were there symptoms?*
    - *Were they diagnosed/treated?*
- Recent travel?
    - *Where?*

ROS:

- Neurologic symptoms?
    - *Possible meningitis, encephalitis, brain abscess*
- Rashes?
    - *Cellulitis, potential systemic infections*
- Focal pain?
    - *Cellulitis, abscess, etc.*
- Resp/GI/GU complaints
    - *Pneumonia, GI illness, UTI/pyelonephritis*

PMH:

- Hx of Alcoholism?
    - *Possible aspiration pneumonia, more susceptible to most types of infections*
- Hx of Cirrhosis?
    - *Possible spontaneous bacterial peritonitis, more susceptible to most types of infections*
- Hx of HIV/AIDs?
    - *Susceptible to certain types of infections (PCP pneumonia, esophageal candidiasis, CMV, Kaposi sarcoma, toxoplasmosis, cryptococcus, cryptosporidiosis, cocci, Histoplasma, mycobacterium avium complex, TB, HSV, etc.)*
- Hx of Diabetes?
    - *More susceptible to pseudomonas infections, but infections in general as well*
- Hx of Cancer?
    - *Immunocompromised state*

Surgical H:

- Recent transplant?
    - *What type of transplant and when?*
- Splenectomy?
    - *Encapsulated organisms (H. influenza type b, strep pneumoniae, N. meningitidis, group B strep, klebsiella, salmonella typhi)*

Social H:

- Alcohol, smoking, recreational drugs, job, living situation, sexual history
- Menstrual history
- Vaccine history

Family H:

Allergies:

Medications:

Physical Examination:

A full exam to look for any signs of infection is warranted. It's important to assess vital signs early as sepsis, severe sepsis, or septic shock will change management and where the patient is admitted to.

- Vital signs
    - Fever, hypotension, tachycardia, hypoxia, signs of SIRS/sepsis
- ABCs
- General appearance
    - Sick or not sick?
- Anxious?
    - Sign of more serious infection

- Agitated?
    - Possible encephalopathy
- Lethargic?
    - Sign of more serious infection
- Full skin exam
    - Look for possible sources of infection, open wounds, abscess, rashes
- Skin tenderness
    - Cellulitis, abscess, necrotizing fasciitis, osteomyelitis
- Mental status exam
    - Infections that may cause encephalopathy
- Nuchal rigidity?
    - Meningitis
- Focal neuro findings?
    - Possible encephalitis or brain abscess

Labs:

- Blood cultures x 2 before antibiotics
- CBC with diff
    - Leukocytosis, neutrophilic shift, neutropenia, anemia
- CMP
    - Elevated LFTs, increased BUN/Cr, electrolyte abnormalities, glucose
- Lactate
    - Lactic acidosis suggestive of infection
- ESR
    - Sign of infection
- CRP
    - Sign of infection
- UA with culture
    - If suspecting UTI
- TSH
- Buffy coat in asplenic patients
- Blood smears if suspecting malaria/babesia/ehrlichiosis
- CSF if possible meningitis (LP)
- Wound cultures
- Procalcitonin

Imaging:

- CT before CSF if have focal findings, change in mental status, papilledema, age >60, immunocompromised
- CXR if indicated

Treatment:

General Treatment:

- Empiric antibiotics is critical right after blood cultures
- Fluids according to sepsis guidelines
- Surgical intervention if needed

- Dexamethasone before antibiotics if suspecting meningitis
- IVIG for toxic shock syndrome and necrotizing fasciitis

Empiric Treatments for Emergency Infections:

Diagnosis	Empiric treatment
Septic shock	Vancomycin Q12h + zosyn 3.375g Q4h
Overwhelming post-splenectomy sepsis	Ceftriaxone 2g Q 12h + vancomycin Q12h
Babesia	Clindamycin 600mg Q8h + quinine 650mg Q8h
Meningococcemia	Ceftriaxone 2g Q12h
Rocky Mountain Spotted Fever	Doxycycline 100mg BID
Toxic Shock Syndrome	Vancomycin + Clindamycin 600mg Q8h
Necrotizing Fasciitis	Vancomycin + Clindamycin 600mg Q8h + meropenem 500mg Q8h, 1g Q8h if suspect pseudomonal infection
Clostridial Myonecrosis	Penicillin 2 million units Q4h + Clindamycin 600mg Q8h
Bacterial Meningitis	Ceftriaxone 2g Q12h + vancomycin + ampicillin if age >55
Brain abscess or suppurative intracranial infection	Vancomycin + Metronidazole 500mg Q8h + Ceftriaxone 2g Q12h
Spinal Epidural Abscess	Vancomycin + Ceftriaxone 2g Q24h
Acute Bacterial Endocarditis	Vancomycin + Ceftriaxone 2g Q12h
Cerebral Malaria	Artesunate 2.4 mg/kg IV at 0, 12, and 24h, then once daily, or quinine IV loading dose of 20mg, then 10mg/kg Q8h

Sepsis Spectrum

Definitions:

Bacteremia- presence of bacteria in blood, as evidenced by positive blood cultures

Systemic Inflammatory Response Syndrome (SIRS)- two or more of the following conditions:

1) **Fever (>38C) or hypothermia (<36C)**
2) **Tachypnea (>24 RR)**
3) **Tachycardia (HR >90)**
4) **Leukocytosis (>12,000), leukopenia (<4,000), or >10% bands**

Sepsis- SIRS + suspected or known infection

Severe sepsis- sepsis + end organ damage displayed by any of the five conditions:

1) **Cardiovascular** (arterial systolic BP ≤ 90 or MAP ≤ 70 that responds to administration of IV fluids)
2) **Renal** (urine output <0.5 ml/kg/hour for 1 hour despite adequate fluid resuscitation)
3) **Respiratory** ($PaO_2/FiO_2 \leq 250$ or if the lung is the only dysfunctional organ ≤ 200)
4) **Hematologic** (platelet count <80,000 or 50% decrease in platelet count from highest value recorded over previous 3 days)
5) **Unexplained metabolic acidosis** (a pH ≤ 7.30 or a base deficit ≥ 5.0 mEq/L and a plasma lactate level > 1.5 times the upper limit of normal for reporting lab)

Septic shock- sepsis with hypotension (<90 or 40 systolic less than the patients normal blood pressure) for **at least 1 hour despite adequate fluid resuscitation**; or the **need for vasopressors to maintain the systolic BP ≥ 90 or MAP ≥ 70**

Refractory septic shock- septic shock that lasts for >1 hour and does not respond to fluid or pressor administration

qSOFA score: scoring system used outside the ICU. ≥ 2 of the following show a poorer prognosis from sepsis **(this is replacing SIRS criteria now for early sepsis identification):**

1) **RR ≥ 22/min**
2) **Altered mentation**
3) **Systolic BP ≤ 100**

History:

There is a wide variation of presentations in people on the sepsis spectrum. Patients can be very ill, yet be afebrile or even hypothermic. Absence of fever is common in neonates, elderly, and patients with uremia or alcoholism. Hyperventilation producing respiratory alkalosis is a common early manifestation of sepsis. There are many different manifestations of sepsis which you should be well familiar with. Many patients will be encephalopathic and will not be able to converse you with you. In these patients, physical exam and correspondence with someone who knows the person is very important.

CC:

HPI:

- COLIDDERRS
- Fever?
  - *Common symptom, part of SIRS criteria*
- Altered mental status?
  - *Maybe a presenting symptom with something as simple as a UTI, but can be many different things, and may show need for intubation*
- Shortness of breath?
  - *Impending respiratory failure possible, possible pneumonia, heart failure*
- Bleeding?
  - *Where from is important*
- Skin changes?
  - *Possible cellulitis, osteomyelitis, gangrene, necrotizing fasciitis, or rashes of various infections*
- Cough?
  - *Possible pneumonia*
- Abdominal pain/swelling?
  - *Possible spontaneous bacterial peritonitis, gastrointestinal infection, cholangitis, cholecystitis, colitis, pancreatitis, etc.*
- N/V?
  - *Able to tolerate PO meds, could be sign of GI infection, and possible hypovolemia*
- Diarrhea/constipation?
  - *Sign of GI infection, and possible hypovolemia*
- Jaundice?
  - *Sign of some sort of hepatobiliary illness*
- Weakness?
  - *Possible respiratory fatigue as well*
- Recent travel?
  - *Infections common to certain areas*

ROS:

PMH:

- Hx of Diabetes?
  - *More prone to infections, and may need to treat hyperglycemia*
- Hx of Recent illness?
  - *What was it?*
  - *How was it treated?*
- Any underlying medical conditions?
  - Two thirds of cases occur in patients with significant underlying disease

Surgical H:

Social H:

- Alcohol, smoking, recreational drugs, job, living situation, sexual history
- Recent travel, recent food consumption

Family H:

Allergies:

Medications:

- Medications, especially new ones should be sought in patients with encephalopathy

Physical:

Vital signs are very important in the physical exam. You should assess the ABC's very quickly as well, as the patient may have an impending loss of their airway due to many causes and may need to be intubated. Once the ABC's are assessed, a full physical exam is warranted. The signs and symptoms of the sepsis spectrum are far too vast to attempt to list here.

- Vital signs
    - See above in definitions for vital signs to look for
- ABC's
- General appearance and mental status
    - May show patient has to be intubated, how toxic they look
- Lymph nodes
    - Signs of infection
- Cranial nerves
    - Look for neurological infections that may have focal neurological signs, like brain abscess, encephalitis, etc.
- Oral mucosa
    - Look for hydration status and possible infectious source
- Neck-stiffness
    - Possible meningitis
- Full cardio exam
    - Murmurs with endocarditis
- Full respiratory exam
    - Pneumonia, CHF, etc.
- Full abdominal exam
    - Tenderness location, source of infection
- Full genital exam
    - UTI, catheter
- Full neuro exam
    - Any focal neurological deficits
- Full integumentary exam
    - Look for any source of infection or rash

Differential:

- Sepsis, severe sepsis, and septic shock implies it is infectious in nature, which is too long to list here as a differential
- Respiratory infections are the most common (64%)
- **Differential of shock (see in ICU basic topics)**

Labs:

- Blood cultures x 2 before antibiotics
- UA with culture
    - Proteinuria, WBCs, glucose, LE, nitrites, etc.
- Sputum culture with gram stain
- CBC with diff
    - Leukocytosis with left shift, thrombocytopenia, leukopenia may develop
- CMP
    - Hyperbilirubinemia, elevated LFTs, abnormal electrolytes, glucose
- Lactate
- Ca
- Mg
- Amylase/lipase
    - May have pancreatitis with infection
- PT/PTT/INR
    - Need to see if a coagulopathy is present
- Thrombin time
- Fibrinogen level
    - Usually decreased
- Arterial blood gas
    - Early stages may see respiratory alkalosis
    - With respiratory fatigue and accumulation of lactate, metabolic acidosis (with increased anion gap) typically supervenes
- Plasma cortisol
    - See if adrenal insufficiency is present
- Cosyntropin test
    - Although, now many experts feel this test is not useful for detecting less profound degrees of corticosteroid deficiency in patients who are critically ill
- Procalcitonin

Imaging:

- EKG
    - May only show sinus tachycardia, may have ST-T wave abnormalities however
- CXR
    - Look for pneumonia or other sources of infection in the chest
- Head CT if encephalopathic
    - Looking for meningitis, encephalitis, brain abscess, head bleeds, etc.
- Others based on patient presentation

- Abdominal CT, MRI of bones/soft tissues, paracentesis in a cirrhotic with ascites, etc.
- Central line
    - For vasopressors and also for invasive monitoring of MAP, CVP, SCVO2, etc.
- Arterial line
    - For continuous monitoring of BP and hemodynamics

Treatment:

Patients with suspected sepsis must be managed urgently. This includes measures to treat the infection (**antibiotics** usually), to provide **hemodynamic and respiratory support**, and to **remove or drain infected tissues**. These measures should be **initiated within one hour of the patient's presentation**.

- **Core principles (from Surviving Sepsis Campaign, Severe Sepsis and Septic Shock, 2016):**
    - Antibiotics within 1 hour of presentation
    - Aggressive early fluid resuscitation (to help prevent getting to septic shock as mortality difference between severe sepsis and septic shock is large)
        - For sepsis induced hypotension, give ≥ 30 mL/kg IV crystalloid fluid in the first 3 hours
        - After initial resuscitation, give additional fluids guided by frequent reassessment of status of hemodynamics like HR, BP, PaO2, RR, temp, UOP, noninvasive (NICOM), and/or invasive monitoring
        - Dynamic over static variables be used to predict fluid responsiveness, where available
        - Target MAP of 65 in patients requiring vasopressors, with norepinephrine as first line therapy, and can add vasopressin to decrease NE dose
        - Guide resuscitation to normalize lactate in those with elevated lactate
    - Source control
- **Clinical trials that were important initially in the management of sepsis spectrum:**
    - **Rivers trial (2001, NEJM)-** (Early goal directed therapy) Among patients with severe sepsis or septic shock, early goal-directed therapy decreases the risk of mortality
        - Used goals of CVP, MAP, ScvO2, and UOP
            - CVP 8-12 mmHg achieved with fluid boluses
            - MAP >65 achieved with vasopressors if needed
            - ScvO2 >70%, achieved with PRBCs and dobutamine if necessary
            - UOP >0.5 mL/kg/hr
        - Now these goals have been shown to not be as beneficial to measure
    - **ProCESS trial (2014, NEJM)-** Among patients with early septic shock, there was no difference in all-cause mortality or in-hospital

mortality at 60 days with management driven by early goal-directed therapy, a novel protocol based therapy, or usual care
- **Antibiotics:**
    - Start as soon as blood and other relevant sites have been obtained for culture
    - **Time to onset of starting antibiotics is a major determinant in the outcome of the patient (start within 1 hour)**
    - Need to have broad gram positive and negative coverage

Patient	Antibiotics
Immunocompetent adult	-Vancomycin 1.5mg/kg Q 12h Plus -Zosyn 3.375 g Q4-6h, OR -Imipenem-cilastin 0.5 g Q 6h or ertapenem 1 g Q 24h, OR -Cefepime 2 g Q 12h
Neutropenic adults (<500 neutrophils/μL)	-Vancomycin 1.5mg/kg Q 12h + -Cefepime 2g Q8h, or -Imipenem-cilastin 0.5 g Q 6h or meropenem 1 g Q 8h, OR -Zosyn 3.375 g Q4-6h + tobramycin 5-7 mg/kg Q 24h
Asplenic patient	-Cefotaxime 2g Q6-8h, OR -Ceftriaxone 2g Q 12h
IV drug user	-Vancomycin 1.5mg/kg Q 12h is **essential**
AIDS patient	-Cefepime 2g Q 8h, OR -Zosyn 3.375g Q 4h + tobramycin 5-7 mg/kg Q 24h

- **Removal of the source of infection:**
    - Sites of occult infection should be sought thoroughly, including the lungs, abdomen, urinary tract, perianal regions, and sacrum
    - Indwelling IV or arterial catheters should be removed, and the tip rolled over a blood agar plate for quantitative culture
        - After antibiotics have been started, a new catheter should be inserted at a different site
    - Foley and drainage catheters should be replaced
    - In patients with severe sepsis arising from the urinary tract, ultrasound or CT should be used to rule out obstruction, perinephric abscess, and renal abscess
    - CT of the abdomen may show evidence of cholecystitis, bile duct dilation, and pus collections
    - Management based off those additional studies
        - Surgery, percutaneous drainage, etc.
- **Hemodynamic, respiratory, and metabolic support:**
    - Primary goals:
        - Restore adequate oxygen and substrate delivery to the tissues
        - Improve tissue oxygen utilization and cellular metabolism
    - Need to maintain adequate organ perfusion

- Circulatory adequacy is assessed by measurement of arterial blood pressure and monitoring of mentation, urinary output, and skin perfusion
- Central venous oxygen saturation CAN be used
  - SCVO2 is often elevated (>75) in septic shock
  - If it is lower than expected, then may have a component of cardiogenic shock
- Management of hypotension:
  - **IV fluids, multiple boluses of NS (be aggressive), then maintenance fluids**
    - For sepsis induced hypotension, give ≥ 30 mL/kg IV crystalloid fluid in the first 3 hours
    - After initial resuscitation, give additional fluids guided by frequent reassessment of status of hemodynamics like HR, BP, PaO2, RR, temp, UOP, noninvasive (NICOM), and/or invasive monitoring
    - Target MAP of 65 in patients requiring vasopressors, with norepinephrine as first line therapy, and can add vasopressin to decrease NE dose
    - Guide resuscitation to normalize lactate in those with elevated lactate
  - Avoid pulmonary edema by maintaining central venous pressure at 8-12
  - Urinary output kept at >0.5 mL/kg/hr
    - A diuretic may be used to maintain this
  - **Maintain MAP of >65 (sys BP >90)**
    - **SEPSISPAM trial (2014, NEJM)-** For patients with septic shock, a goal MAP of 80-85 does not reduce all-cause mortality at 28 days when compared to a goal of 65-70. The higher MAP goal was associated with reduction in rates of renal dysfunction for patients with a history of chronic hypertension
  - **Norepinephrine** may be used if MAP of >65 cannot be met only after aggressive fluid resuscitation, also if sys BP <70
  - Can used **vasopressin** as an adjunct to NE to down-titrate NE dose
    - **VASST trial (2008, NEJM)-** Among patients with septic shock on a catecholamine vasopressor, addition of low-dose vasopressin did not reduce all-cause mortality at 28 days when compared to addition of NE
  - If myocardial dysfunction produces elevated cardiac pressure and low CO, dobutamine may be used (sys BP >100 and normal diastolic BP), dopamine also (sys BP 70-100 and bradycardic)
    - **SOAP II trial (2010, NEJM)-** In the treatment of shock, norepinephrine and dopamine compare similarly with respect to

28-day mortality, but dopamine is associated with an increased risk of arrhythmia
- Can use **NICOM** machine to help say if hypotension is fluid responsive or not (passive leg raising)
  - Assess SV variation with passive leg raising
  - If SV variation is ≥10%, then patient is fluid responsive, and boluses should be given
- Albumin has NOT been shown to show any mortality benefit
  - **ALBIOS trial (2014, NEJM)-** Among patients with severe sepsis or septic shock, daily administration of albumin to maintain serum albumin ≥3 g/dL was not associated with a reduction in all-cause mortality at 28 days when compared to no albumin

- Adrenal insufficiency:
  - Critical illness-related corticosteroid insufficiency (CIRCI) should be considered in someone whose hypotension does not improve with fluid replacement therapy
  - **Hydrocortisone** 50mg IV Q6h should be given if fail fluids and vasopressors
    - Hastens recovery from sepsis-induced hypotension without increasing long-term survival
    - Does NOT help to prevent severe sepsis from escalating into septic shock
  - **CORTICUS trial (2008, NEJM)-** Hydrocortisone hastens the reversal of shock but does not confer a survival benefit among patients with septic shock
  - **HYPRESS trial (2016, JAMA)-** In patients with severe sepsis, hydrocortisone therapy does not reduce the progression to septic shock at 14 days compared to placebo. Hydrocortisone therapy also failed to result in improvement from time to septic shock or intermediate term mortality. Hydrocortisone was associated with a 10% absolute increase in hyperglycemia and an absolute 13% reduction in delirium.

- Anemia:
  - Unless actively bleeding, transfusion threshold should be <7
  - **TRISS trial (2014, NEJM)-** Patients with septic shock who underwent transfusion at a Hgb threshold of 7 had similar mortality at 90 days but used 50% fewer units of blood compared with those who underwent transfusion at a Hgb threshold of 9

- Respiratory support:
  - **Ventilator therapy indications:**
    - Progressive hypoxemia
    - Progressive hypercapnia
    - Neurologic deterioration
    - Respiratory muscle failure
  - Sustained tachypnea (RR ≥ 30/min) is frequently a sign of impending respiratory failure

- Ventilation is initiated to deliver adequate oxygen to tissues, to divert blood from muscles of respiration to other organs, prevent oropharyngeal aspiration, and to reduce cardiac afterload
- **Use low tidal volumes (6-8 mL/kg of ideal body weight)**
- Careful sedation with daily sedation holidays
- Elevation of the head of the bed
- Stress ulcer prophylaxis with H2 blockers to prevent GI hemorrhage in ventilated patients
  - Other metabolic therapy:
    - Transfusion:
      - Erythrocyte transfusion generally recommended at hemoglobin ≤ 7, with a target of 9
      - FFP, platelets, cryoprecipitate for DIC
    - Bicarbonate:
      - Sometimes administered for severe metabolic acidosis (arterial pH < 7.2) as vasopressors do not work as well with low pH

- **General support:**
  - Nutritional supplementation
  - Only use insulin if needed to maintain glucose concentration below 144-180 mg/dL
    - May need to give dextrose as fluids if have poor nutrition in addition to insulin, even though that is counterintuitive
  - Can do an insulin drip to maintain levels in appropriate range
  - Endotoxin-neutralizing proteins, COX inhibitors, NO synthase inhibitors, anticoagulants, polyclonal immunoglobulins, glucocorticoids, phospholipid emulsion, activated protein C, and antagonists to TNF-alpha, IL-1, platelet-activating factor, and bradykinin have all been shown to **NOT** improve rates of survival

- **Prophylaxis in the ICU:**
  - Stress ulcer prophylaxis:
    - Use H2 blockers (less side effects)
    - Use PPIs if have coagulopathy or are bleeding
    - Nutrition
  - DVT prophylaxis:
    - Heparin, lovenox, SCDs, **walking** (if possible)
  - Ventilator associated prophylaxis:
    - Prevention of aspiration by elevating head of bed >30 degrees for at least 18 hours a day
    - Suctioning mouth when needed and other oral care
    - Daily weaning trials
    - Humidifier
  - Delirium prophylaxis:
    - Open shades during day, reduce sedation when possible, familiarize patient room
  - Muscle fatigue prophylaxis:
    - Get patient out of bed early
    - Start PT when able
  - Decubitus ulcer prophylaxis:
    - Turn patient several times a day, skin care, flotation bed, etc.

- Aspiration precautions:
  - Elevated head of bed >30 degrees for at least 18 hours a day, suctioning when needed

Etiology:

- Blood cultures only produce bacteria or fungi in ~20-40% of cases of severe sepsis, and ~40-70% of cases of septic shock
- Respiratory infection is the most common cause (64%)
- 62% are gram negative bacteria (pseudomonas and E. coli most common)
- 47% were gram positive (S. aureus most common)
- 19% were fungi (Candida species most common)

Risk Factors:

- Infection of any source
- Infants
- Elderly
- Diabetes
- Cancer
- Immunocompromised

Pathogenesis:

- **General overview:**
  - There are many different mechanisms of the pathophysiology of sepsis
  - Starts with an infectious source and triggers host defenses
  - All the mechanisms of sepsis pathophysiology are not worked out
- **Host mechanisms for sensing microbes:**
  - Recognition of lipid A of LPS
  - LPS binding protein transfers LPS to CD14, to toll like receptor 4, which transduces a signal to the interior of the cell
  - TNF then amplifies that signal
  - Many different factors then come into play to begin the host defense mechanism
- **Local and systemic host responses to invading microbes:**
  - Cytokines, chemokines, prostanoids, leukotrienes, and others are released to increased blood flow to the infected area **(rubor)**, enhance the permeability of local blood vessels **(tumor)**, recruit neutrophils and other cells **(calor)**, and elicit pain **(dolor)**
  - Local inflammation occurs
  - TNF alpha stimulates leukocytes and vascular endothelial cells to release other cytokines, express surface cell molecules that enhance neutrophil recruitment, and increase prostaglandin and leukotriene production
  - Intravascular thrombosis occurs as a part of the local inflammatory response
  - IL-6 promotes intravascular coagulation
  - Tissue factor is expressed, which binds factor VIIa to activate X and IX into their enzymatically active forms

- Clotting is also favored by impaired function of protein C/S, and depletion of antithrombin and proteins C/S
- Neutrophil extracellular traps (NETs) are produced, and release granule proteins and chromatin
- NETs kill bacteria and fungi with elastase and histones
- IL-6 plays an important role in the systemic compartment by stimulating the hypothalamic-pituitary-adrenal axis, by being a major procoagulant cytokine, and is a principal inducer of the acute phase response

- **Organ dysfunction and shock:**
  - **Endothelial injury** occurs
    - The endothelium is important for regulating vascular tone, vascular permeability, and coagulation
    - TNF alpha induces vascular endothelial cells to produce and release cytokines, procoagulant molecules, platelet activating factor, NO, and other mediators
      - When endothelial injury, these will not operate as well as it should
    - Tissue oxygenation may decrease as the number of functioning capillaries decreases by luminal obstruction due to swollen endothelial cells, decreased deformability of circulating erythrocytes, leukocyte platelet-fibrin thrombi, or compression by edema fluid
    - Local accumulation of lactic acid occurs as oxygenation decreases
  - **Septic shock:**
    - Hallmark of septic shock is a decrease in peripheral vascular resistance that occurs despite increased levels of vasopressor catecholamines
    - Blood lactate levels increase as oxygen delivery is depressed to tissues
    - Central venous oxygen saturation becomes high

Complications:

- **Cardiopulmonary complications:**
  - Ventilation perfusion mismatching produces a fall in arterial PO2 early in the course
  - Increasing alveolar epithelial injury and permeability results in increased pulmonary water content, decreased compliance, and interferes with O2 exchange
  - **ARDS can occur:**
    - In the absence of pneumonia or heart failure, progressive diffuse pulmonary infiltrates and arterial hypoxemia occurring within 1 week of known insult indicate development of ARDS **(PaO2/FiO2 200-300)**
    - This occurs in ~50% of patients with severe sepsis or septic shock
  - Elevated PCWP (>18) suggests fluid volume overload or cardiac failure rather than ARDS
  - **Hypotension:**

- Usually results initially from maldistribution of blood flow and blood volume from hypovolemia from diffuse capillary leakage of intravascular fluid
- Dehydration, vomiting, diarrhea, hemorrhage, polyuria, etc. may contribute
- Initially have elevated SVR and decreased CO
- Later in the course, get normal or increased CO with decreased SVR
  - This distinguishes sepsis hypotension from cardiogenic, extracardiac obstructive, and hypovolemic shock
  - **Depression of myocardial function:**
    - Increased end diastolic and systolic ventricular volumes with decreased EF develops within 24 hours in most patients with severe sepsis

- **Adrenal insufficiency:**
  - May be very difficult to diagnose
  - Cosyntropin test not very useful anymore
  - Critical illness-related corticosteroid insufficiency (CIRCI) occurs, which was proposed to encompass the different mechanisms that may produce corticosteroid activity that is inadequate for the severity of the patients illness
  - May be from structural damage to the adrenal gland, but is **more commonly due to reversible dysfunction of the hypothalamic-pituitary axis or to tissue corticosteroid resistance** resulting from abnormalities of the glucocorticoid receptor or increased conversion of cortisol to cortisone
  - **Refractory hypotension** is the major clinical manifestation of CIRCI
  - Hyponatremia and hyperkalemia are actually usually absent
  - Eosinophilia and hypoglycemia may be present

- **Renal complications:**
  - Oliguria, azotemia, proteinuria, and non-specific urinary casts are frequently seen
  - Many are inappropriately polyuric, which may be exacerbated by hyperglycemia
  - Most renal failure in sepsis is due to **acute tubular necrosis** induced by **hypovolemia, arterial hypotension, or toxic drugs**

- **Coagulopathy:**
  - Thrombocytopenia (10-30% of patients)
  - Platelets are very low in patients with DIC (<50,000)

- **Neurologic complications:**
  - Delirium (acute encephalopathy) is often an early manifestation of sepsis (occurs in 10-70% of patients at some point during the hospital stay)
  - If sepsis lasts for weeks to months, 'critical illness' polyneuropathy may prevent weaning from ventilatory support and produce distal muscle weakness
  - Long term cognitive loss has been documented in survivors of severe sepsis

- **Immunosuppression:**
  - Common

- Loss of delayed type hypersensitivity reactions, failure to control the primary infection, increased risk for secondary infection (ie from opportunistic infections)
- ~1/3 of patients experience reactivation of HSV, varicella, or CMV

Admission Orders:

- Admit to ICU
- Diagnosis severe sepsis or septic shock
- Condition critical
- Vital signs every 15 minutes X 4 hours, then hourly if stable, call for BP < 90/60, HR > 120, worsening oxygenation, urinary output < 30 mL/h
- Allergies
- Activity bedrest
- Nursing foley catheter, strict I/O's, daily weights, neurologic checks Q2h, call for worsening neurologic status
- Diet NPO
- Fluids sepsis resuscitation
- Meds:
    - Vancomycin 1g IV Q12h
    - Zosyn 3.375 g Q4-6h
    - Insulin drip per ICU protocol, to maintain blood glucose 144-180 mg/dL
    - Vasopressors if needed
    - H2 blocker of choice
    - Hydrocortisone 50mg IV Q6h if refractory hypotension to fluids and pressors
    - Heparin 5000 units SubQ Q8h
- Labs/diagnostics:
    - On admission:
        - Blood cultures x 2, UA with culture, sputum culture
        - CBC with diff and plt count
        - CMP
        - Ca
        - Mg
        - LFTs
        - Amylase
        - PT/PTT/INR
        - Thrombin time
        - Fibrinogen level
        - Lactate
        - ABG
        - EKG
        - CXR
    - Daily:
        - CBC with diff
        - CMP
        - Ca
        - Mg
        - PT/PTT/INR

Discharge Information:

- Will discharge to the floor, never from ICU to home
- Daily communication between ICU care team and patients family can help define the goals of care and ensure decisions are made in the patients best interest

Additional Notes:

- Important clinical trials:
    - **Surviving Sepsis Campaign (see online)**
    - **Rivers trial (2001, NEJM)-** Among patients with severe sepsis or septic shock, early goal-directed therapy decreases the risk of mortality
        - Used goals of CVP, MAP, ScvO2, and UOP
            - CVP 8-12 mmHg achieved with fluid boluses
            - MAP >65 achieved with vasopressors if needed
            - ScvO2 >70%, achieved with PRBCs and dobutamine if necessary
            - UOP >0.5 mL/kg/hr
        - Now these goals have been shown to **not** be as beneficial to measure
    - **ProCESS trial (2014, NEJM)-** Among patients with early septic shock, there was no difference in all-cause mortality in-hospital mortality at 60 days with management driven by early goal-directed therapy, a novel protocol based therapy, or usual care
    - **SEPSISPAM trial (2014, NEJM)-** For patients with septic shock, a goal MAP of 80-85 does not reduce all-cause mortality at 28 days when compared to a goal of 65-70. The higher MAP goal was associated with reduction in rates of renal dysfunction for patients with a history of chronic hypertension
    - **VASST trial (2008, NEJM)-** Among patients with septic shock on a catecholamine vasopressor, addition of low-dose vasopressin did not reduce all-cause mortality at 28 days when compared to addition of NE
    - **SOAP II trial (2010, NEJM)-** In the treatment of shock, norepinephrine and dopamine compare similarly with respect to 28-day mortality, but dopamine is associated with an increased risk of arrhythmia
    - **ALBIOS trial (2014, NEJM)-** Among patients with severe sepsis or septic shock, daily administration of albumin to maintain serum albumin $\geq$3 g/dL was not associated with a reduction in all-cause mortality at 28 days when compared to no albumin
    - **CORTICUS trial (2008, NEJM)-** Hydrocortisone hastens the reversal of shock but does not confer a survival benefit among patients with septic shock
    - **HYPRESS trial (2016, JAMA)-** In patients with severe sepsis, hydrocortisone therapy does not reduce the progression to septic shock at 14 days compared to placebo. Hydrocortisone therapy also failed to result in improvement from time to septic shock or intermediate term mortality. Hydrocortisone was associated with a

10% absolute increase in hyperglycemia and an absolute 13% reduction in delirium.
- **TRISS trial (2014, NEJM)-** Patients with septic shock who underwent transfusion at a Hgb threshold of 7 had similar mortality at 90 days but used 50% fewer units of blood compared with those who underwent transfusion at a Hgb threshold of 9

Infectious Endocarditis

Definitions:

Endocarditis- infection of the endothelium of the heart (not limited to valves)

Acute bacterial endocarditis (ABE)- infection of normal valves with virulent organisms (s. aureus, group A or other beta-hemolytic streptococci, strep pneumoniae)

Subacute bacterial endocarditis (SBE)- indolent infection with less virulent organisms (s. viridians) often on abnormal valves

History:

Endocarditis is very difficult to diagnose, especially if you do not have a clinical suspicion. 80-90% of people have a fever, with chills and sweats as the second most common symptom at 40-75%. In someone with a fever and a murmur (new or old), endocarditis should be on the differential. It is important to know if the murmur is new or not, but it should be ruled out no matter what.

CC:

HPI:

- COLIDDERRS
- Fever?
  - *Part of Dukes criteria, minor*
- Chills?
  - *Common symptom of endocarditis*
- Prior endocarditis?
  - *Major risk factor, Dukes criteria, minor*
- Weight loss/anorexia?
  - *Common symptom*
- Myalgias?
  - *Can have myalgias, not part of Dukes criteria*
- Nail changes?
  - *Splinter hemorrhages may be present, not part of Dukes criteria*
- Skin changes?
  - *Janeway lesions (painless erythematous lesions on palms/soles) Dukes criteria, minor*
  - *Oslers nodes (painful raised lesions on fingers, toes, or feet) Dukes criteria, minor*
- Recent travel?
  - *Certain infectious causes*
- Arthritis?
  - *Can have joint pain, not part of Dukes criteria*
- Hematuria?
  - *Can have glomerulonephritis with endocarditis, Dukes criteria, minor*
- Stroke symptoms?

- Can have septic emboli or intracranial hemorrhage, Dukes criteria, minor
- Vision changes?
  - Can have Roth spots (oval, retinal hemorrhages with a clear, pale center) that can cause vision changes, Dukes criteria, minor

ROS:

PMH:

- Hx of Endocarditis?
  - *Risk factor for current endocarditis and Dukes criteria, minor*
- Hx of Valvular disease/murmur?
  - *Helps if you notice a murmur to know if they had one previously or not, and aortic valve disease is a Dukes criteria, minor*
- Hx of Rheumatic fever?
  - *Rheumatic valve disease is a Dukes criteria, minor*

Surgical H:

- Recent surgeries (cardiac procedures with grafts, pacemakers)?
  - *Important as this will change treatment*

Social H:

- Alcohol, smoking, **recreational drugs (IV),** job, living situation, sexual history

Family H:

Allergies:

Medications:

Physical Examination:

There are specific physical exam findings that should be looked for in suspected endocarditis (bolded below). Although these findings are rare, they are a part of the Dukes criteria, and should be looked for. It's important to assess vital signs and overall toxicity of the patient.

- Vital signs
  - Fever is a Dukes minor criteria, look for tachycardia, signs of sepsis
- **Roth spots** (retinal hemorrhages + pale center, immunologic)?
  - Dukes criteria, minor
- Petechiae?
- Cardiac
  - Murmur? Worsening murmur? Friction rub?
    - Murmur in person with fever need to suspect endocarditis
  - Thrill, S3/4
  - Conduction defects
    - Endocarditis can cause arrhythmias

- Respiratory
- Abdomen
    - Splenomegaly (splenic abscess is a complication of endocarditis)
- Musculoskeletal pain
- **Janeway lesions** (non-tender hemorrhagic macules on palms/soles, caused by septic emboli)
    - Dukes minor criteria
- **Oslers nodes** (tender nodules on pads of digits, caused by immune complex deposition)
    - Dukes minor criteria
- **Nail bed splinter hemorrhages**
- Clubbing
- Mental status
    - Can have septic emboli to the brain
- Tenderness at pacemaker site if present
    - Sign of endocarditis with pacemaker involvement which changes treatment
- Full neuro exam

Differential Diagnosis:

- Valvular abnormality with no endocarditis (ie rheumatic heart disease, mitral valve prolapse, bicuspid/calcific aortic valve)
    - *Murmur without other signs/symptoms of endocarditis*
- Flow murmur (anemia, pregnancy, hyperthyroidism, sepsis high stress state)
    - *Murmur without other signs/symptoms of endocarditis, plus other signs of the disease causing the flow murmur*
- Atrial myxoma
    - *Possible murmur, but no fever, DOE, PND, orthopnea, may mimic right or left sided heart failure*
- Non-infective endocarditis (Libmann-sacks in SLE)
    - *Murmur, possible fever, symptoms of SLE*
- Marantic endocarditis (NBTE)
    - *Possible CVA, CHF symptoms, etc.*
- Hematuria if present due to other causes (glomerulonephritis, renal cell carcinoma)
    - *Elevated BUN/Cr with no other symptoms of endocarditis*
- Acute renal failure
    - *Azotemia with no other symptoms of endocarditis*
- Vasculitis
    - *Can have systemic symptoms, but usually no murmur*

Labs:

- Blood cultures (2 sets from different site) every day until negative
    - Look for S. aureus, strep viridians, enterococcus, S. epidermidis, HACEK organisms
    - Dukes criteria, major
- CBC with diff
    - Leukocytosis, anemia, neutrophilic shift, etc.
- CMP

- Look for elevated BUN/Cr, electrolyte abnormalities, elevated LFTs, glucose
- ESR
  - Commonly elevated in endocarditis
- CRP
  - Commonly elevated in endocarditis
- Lactate
  - Lactic acidosis common
- Circulating immune complex titer
  - For glomerulonephritis
- Rheumatoid factor
  - Can be elevated in endocarditis

Imaging:

- EKG
  - Check for arrhythmias, ischemia, LVH, etc.
- PA/Lat CXR
  - Looking for signs of cardiac abnormalities, can have lung abnormalities from septic pulmonary emboli, also ruling out other abnormalities in the chest
- TTE if low clinical suspicion
  - Low suspicion if 1 major and 1 minor, or 3 minor
- TEE if high clinical suspicion
  - High suspicion if two major, one major and 3 minor, or 5 minor

Dukes Criteria:

Used to diagnose endocarditis. Separated into major and minor criteria. To diagnose, need either 2 major, 1 major + 3 minor, or 5 minor criteria.

- **Major criteria:**
  - Sustained bacteremia by a bacteria known to cause endocarditis, or 1+ blood culture from Coxiella
  - Endocardial involvement seen by echo
  - NEW valvular regurgitation seen by echo
- **Minor criteria:**
  - Predisposing condition:
    - Previous endocarditis
    - Rheumatic valve disease
    - Aortic valve disease
    - Complex cyanotic heart lesion
    - Prosthesis
    - IV drug abuse
  - Fever ($\geq$ 38C or $\geq$ 100.4F)
  - Vascular phenomena:
    - Major arterial emboli
    - Septic pulmonary infarcts
    - Mycotic aneurysm
    - Intracranial hemorrhage
    - Conjunctival hemorrhages

- Janeway lesions (painless erythematous lesions on palms/soles)
    - Immunologic phenomena:
        - Glomerulonephritis
        - Oslers nodes (painful, raised lesions on fingers, toes, or feet)
        - Roth spots (oval, retinal hemorrhages with a clear pale center)
        - Rheumatoid factor
    - Microbiologic evidence:
        - + blood culture but not meeting major criteria

Treatment:

- If ABE, start empiric treatment promptly after 2 culture data obtained
- If SBE, and if hemodynamically stable, delay antibiotics until culture results come back, if unstable start empiric treatment
- **Empiric treatment:**
    - Native valve ABE:
        - Vancomycin IV 15mg/kg Q 8-12h + ceftriaxone or gentamicin
    - Native valve SBE:
        - Ceftriaxone 1-2g IM/IV Q24h
        - Doxycycline if want Bartonella coverage
    - Prosthetic valve endocarditis:
        - If prosthesis in place for < 1 year:
            - Ceftriaxone 1-2g Q24h +
            - Gentamicin 1-1.7 kg/mg IM/IV Q8h +
            - Cefepime 1-2g IV Q12h +
            - Rifampin 300mg PO Q8h x 6 weeks
        - If prosthesis in place for ≥ 1 year:
            - Same as native valve SBE
- **Tailor specific therapies once culture susceptibilities come back**
- If cardiovascular implantable electronic devices are in place:
    - Remove the device
    - 4-6 weeks of antibiotics
- **Indications for surgery:**
    - CHF due to new or worsening valvular disease
    - Perivalvular infection
    - Partially dehisced unstable prosthetic device
    - Left sided endocarditis caused by staphylococcus aureus, fungal, or other highly resistant organisms
    - Endocarditis complicated by heart block, annular or aortic abscess, or destructive penetrating lesion
    - Persistent bacteremia or fever lasting 5-7 days after starting antibiotic therapy
    - Cardiovascular implantable electronic device endocarditis
    - Early surgery (within 48 hours after diagnosis) in patients with large vegetations (>10mm)
        - **EASE trial (2012, NEJM)-** Reduced embolic events but had similar in-hospital and 6 month mortality rated compared to delayed surgery

Etiology:

- **IV drug abuse – S. aureus, pseudomonas, candida → tricuspid valve and pulmonary septic emboli**
- **Dental procedures- strep viridians (most common cause for left sided SBE)**
- **Prosthetic valve- S. aureus and s. epidermidis**
- **GI malignancy- strep gallolyticus (bovis)**
- **Nosocomial UTI- enterococcus**
- **Culture negative- antibiotics before cultures, HACEK, Coxiella, Bartonella, Brucella**
- S. viridians, enterococcus, coxiella, S. aureus, S. epidermidis, HACEK (haemophilus, Aggregatibacter, actinomycelemocomitans, cardiobacterim, Eikenella, Kingella), strep bovis (gallolyticus)

Risk Factors:

- IV drug abuse
    - Usually right sided endocarditis, can have pulmonary septic emboli, usually from staph aureus, very sick in appearance
- Indwelling venous catheter
- Poor dentition
- Hemodialysis
- Diabetes
- Pacemaker
- ICD
- Also see section of indications for prophylaxis

Pathogenesis:

- **Endothelial injury** allows either direct infection by virulent organisms or platelet-fibrin thrombus development (NBTE, SLE)
- Organisms enter blood stream through mucosa, skin, or sites of local infection, and latch onto platelet-fibrin thrombus or injured endothelium
- Adhesin molecules on the bacteria (MSCRAMM's) adhere to NBTE or injured endothelium
- Fibronectin-binding proteins, clumping factor, etc act on site
- **Fibrin deposition combines with platelet aggregation and organism proliferation to cause a vegetation**
- **Organisms deep in the vegetation are non-growing and relatively resistant to antibiotics, while surface organisms proliferate and release organisms into the blood stream**
- Cytokine production → fever
- Embolization of vegetations → stroke, pulmonary infarcts, Janeway lesions
- Tissue injury from circulating immune complexes or immune responses to deposited bacterial antigens

Complications:

- CHF
- **Conduction defects**
- Stroke

- Cerebral aneurysm
- Mycotic aneurysm
- **Perivalvular abscess**
- Pericarditis
- Systemic emboli (pulmonary, kidney, spleen, brain)
- Glomerulonephritis
- **Splenic abscess**
- Meningitis

Prophylaxis for Endocarditis:

- **Indications for endocarditis prophylaxis:**
    - Prosthetic heart valves
    - Prior endocarditis
    - Unrepaired cyanotic congenital heart disease, including palliative shunts or conduits
    - Incompletely repaired congenital heart disease with residual defects adjacent to prosthetic material
    - Valvulopathy developing after cardiac transplantation
    - **Notice mitral valve prolapse is NOT an indication anymore**, neither is rheumatic heart disease or bicuspid aortic valve
- Treatment:
    - Only HIGH risk procedures need prophylaxis
        - Dental manipulation of gingival tissue or periapical region of teeth or perforation of oral mucosa
        - Respiratory tract procedures with incision or biopsy, tonsillectomy, adenoidectomy
        - Procedures in patients with ongoing GI/GU tract infection or infected skin or musculoskeletal tissue
        - Cardiac surgery
    - LOW risk procedures do NOT need prophylaxis
        - GI procedures (ERCP, EGD)
        - GU procedures (prostatectomy, catheter insertions)
        - Vaginal or cesarean delivery
    - Standard PO- **amoxicillin** 2g PO 1h before procedure
    - Cannot do PO- ampicillin 2g IV within 1h before procedure
    - Penicillin allergy- clarithromycin, azithromycin, cephalexin, or clindamycin
    - Penicillin allergy but cannot do PO- ceftriaxone, cefazolin, or clindamycin

Admission Orders:

- Admit to telemetry
- Diagnosis bacterial endocarditis
- Condition serious
- Vital signs Temp, BP, HR, RR, and O2 saturation Q4h until afebrile for 24h, then per routine
- Allergies
- Activity as tolerated
- Nursing daily weights, strict I's/O's
- Diet regular

- Fluids sepsis resuscitation
- Meds:
    - Tylenol 325-650mg PO Q4-6h prn
    - Empiric antibiotic therapy (see earlier)
- Labs/diagnostics:
    - Blood cultures X2 before antibiotics
    - CBC with diff
    - CMP
    - UA
    - PA/lat CXR
    - EKG
    - TEE or TTE based on clinical suspicion
    - Daily CBC until WBC count normal
- Infectious disease and cardiac surgery consult

Discharge Information:

- Plan for possibility of prolonged IV antibiotics (4-6 weeks) if endocarditis is confirmed
    - Options are home IV infusion
    - Outpatient IV antibiotics at infusion center
    - Nursing home placement

Additional Notes:

- Important clinical trials:
    - **EASE trial (2012, NEJM)-** Reduced embolic events but had similar in-hospital and 6 month mortality rated compared to delayed surgery

Acute Bacterial/Aseptic Meningitis

Definitions:

Bacterial meningitis- bacterial infection of the subarachnoid space

Aseptic meningitis- negative bacterial microbiological data. CSF pleocytosis with negative appropriate blood and CSF cultures. Aseptic less likely to be bacterial but can be infectious or non-infectious.

History:

The typical triad of headache, fever, and nuchal rigidity only occurs in 44% of meningitis patients. This means it is important to look for risk factors of meningitis, as well as having a high clinical suspicion if any typical meningitis signs are present. Subacute meningitis may be more subtle, which should be investigated thoroughly if the person is immunocompromised (like HIV infection with Cryptococcus meningitis).

CC:

HPI:

- COLIDDERRS
    - *Meningitis presents with fever, headache, and a stiff neck*
    - *Encephalitis presents with fever, headache, and altered mental status*
    - *Brain abscess presents with fever, headache, and focal neurological deficits*
- Change in mental status?
    - *Less suggestive of meningitis and more towards encephalitis, but doesn't rule out meningitis*
- Headache?
    - *Common symptom*
- Fever?
    - *Common symptom*
- Nuchal rigidity?
    - *Common symptom*
- Acuteness of symptoms?
    - *More subacute symptoms can indicate infections like Cryptococcus or toxoplasmosis in an immunocompromised host (like HIV/AIDS)*
- N/V?
    - *Can be a sign of increased intracranial pressure in abscess*
- Photophobia?
    - *Common symptom of meningitis, but can also be in migraine*
- Recent illness (sinusitis, otitis media, mononucleosis)?
    - *These infections can lead to meningitis*
- Loss of lateral eye movements?
    - *Can occur in meningitis, but also any brain infections*
- Weakness?

- Rash?
  - *Looking for meningococcus rash, RMSF, etc.*
- Hiking recently?
  - *RMSF, Human granulocytic ehrlichiosis, Human monocytic ehrlichiosis*
- Tick bites?
  - *RMSF, Human granulocytic ehrlichiosis, Human monocytic ehrlichiosis*
- Cat litter box exposure?
  - *Toxoplasmosis*
- Pigeon droppings exposure?
  - *Cryptococcus*

  - *Focal neurological deficits more likely brain abscess, but can occur in meningitis, encephalitis, brain abscess, etc.*

ROS:

PMH:

- Hx of Diabetes?
  - *Makes them more susceptible to infections*
- Hx of TB?
  - *Can have disseminated secondary TB to meningitis*
- Hx of HIV?
  - *Cryptococcus, toxoplasmosis, etc.*
- Hx of Complement deficiency?
  - *Neisseria meningitis*
- Hx of SLE?
  - *Can cause neurological symptoms*
- Hx of Sarcoidosis?
  - *Can cause neurological symptoms*
- Hx of Herpes?
  - *HSV is a common cause viral meningitis*
- Hx of Syphilis?
  - *Can cause neurological symptoms*

Surgical H:

- Splenectomy?
  - *Makes them susceptible to encapsulated organisms, like Neisseria meningitis*
- Neurological surgeries?
  - *Leaves them susceptible to certain infections like S. aureus, coagulase negative staph, pseudomonas, E. coli, and Acinetobacter baumannii*

Social H:

- Alcohol, smoking, recreational drugs, job, living situation, sexual history
- **Vaccinations for strep pneumoniae, MMR, and H. influenza**
- Recent travel?

Family H:

Allergies:

Medications:

Physical Examination:

Vital signs and how toxic the patient appears is important in the physical exam. Since meningococcal meningitis is acutely life threatening, look for the typical petechial rash that occurs in younger patients. A full neuro exam is important.

- Vital signs
    - Fever, tachycardia, SaO2, etc.
- Mental status
    - Altered more likely suggestive of encephalitis or brain abscess than meningitis
- GCS
    - May need to intubate the patient if altered enough if they can't protect their airway
- Nuchal rigidity
    - **Kernigs sign** → supine with knees flexed, then extend the legs and neck will flex
    - **Brudzinski's sign** → supine, flex neck, knees will bend
    - Not very reliable, if negative it means nothing
- Eye exam
    - Can have loss of lateral eye movements
- CN's
    - Look for focal neurological deficits
- Full neuro with DTRs and strength
    - Look for focal neurological deficits
- Skin exam
    - Looking for rashes that may suggest the etiology (Neisseria meningitidis, RMSF, etc.)
- Respiratory
- Cardiac
    - Can have a concurrent endocarditis with strep pneumoniae (Osler's triad- Meningitis + pneumoniae + endocarditis)
- Mouth/genital exam for herpes outbreak

Differential Diagnosis:

- Bacterial meningitis differential:
    - Encephalitis (particularly HSV)
        - *Can present with classic meningitis symptoms, may have history of HSV, primarily affects the temporal lobes of the brain*
    - Rocky Mountain Spotted Fever
        - *Endemic to east coast, wood tick, fever, headache, rash that starts on wrist and ankle then migrates to trunk, thrombocytopenia, hyponatremia, and elevated LFTs*
    - Human granulocytic/monocytic ehrlichiosis

- *Tick bite exposure with myalgias, headache, fever, rash is rare*
- Subarachnoid hemorrhage
  - *No fever, younger person with thunderclap headache*
- Brain abscess
  - *Fever, headache, focal neurological symptoms, possible infection that preceded this*
- Brain tumor
  - *No fever, headache, n/v, possible cancer history that has now metastasized, B-symptoms*
- Sarcoidosis
  - *Neurological symptoms that also has typical sarcoidosis findings (black female, uveitis, interstitial fibrosis, erythema nodosum, lupus pernio (frost bite appearance))*
- SLE
  - *Neurological symptoms with typical symptoms of SLE (young female, malar rash, discoid rash, mucositis, serositis, arthritis, renal disorders, photosensitivity, hematologic disorders)*
- Behcet's syndrome
  - *Neurological manifestations can be a late manifest but usually have recurrent painful genital ulcers/apthous ulcer and uveitis*
- Vogt-Koyanagi-Harada syndrome
  - *Can have meningitis symptoms with ocular problems, sudden loss of vision, ocular pain, and photophobia*
- Subacute/chronic meningitis
  - *More subtle symptoms, most likely immunocompromised, different microbiological sources*
- Dural sinus thrombosis
  - *No fever, headache, possibly focal neurological symptoms, CT findings*
- Thrombotic thrombocytopenic purpura
  - *Fever, anemia, thrombocytopenia, renal failure, neurological symptoms*
- Febrile seizure
  - *Younger patient with seizure like activity and fever*
- Amebic meningoencephalitis
  - *High fever, headache, stiff neck, n/v, child or young adult, possibly went swimming or was in water*

- Aseptic (viral) meningitis differential:
  - Untreated or partially treated bacterial meningitis
    - *History of meningitis that wasn't treated properly or antibiotics were not completed*
  - Fungal/mycobacteria/neurosyphylis
    - *Typical symptoms depends on the cause*
  - Mycoplasma
    - *Can have erythema multiforme, possible pneumonia that lead to meningitis*
  - Listeria
    - *Can affect infants, immunocompromised, pregnant women, see meningitis, monocytes in the CSF*
  - Brucella

- *Unpasteurized milk or goat cheese, lymphadenopathy with granulomas, undulating fever*
  - Coxiella
    - *Cattle placenta, Q fever, pneumonia, no rash*
  - Leptospira
    - *Headache, fever, muscle pain usually in the calf and lumbar areas, pharyngitis, nonpruritic skin rash*
  - Rickettsia
    - *Fever, headache, rash, arthropod vector*
  - Parameningeal infections
    - *Depends on what is causing it*
  - Neoplastic
    - *No fever, headache, n/v, possible history of cancer with metastasis*
  - SLE
    - *See above*
  - Sarcoidosis
    - *See above*
  - Behcet's syndrome
    - *See above*

Labs:

- For suspected bacterial:
  - **Blood cultures x 2 (then dexamethasone, then empiric antibiotics)**
  - Lumbar puncture (opening pressure, WBC count, RBC count, glucose, CSF/serum glucose, protein, gram stain, culture, latex agglutination, PCR)
    - *See chart below for CSF findings and their meanings*
  - CBC with diff
    - *Look for leukocytosis, anemia, thrombocytopenia, neutrophilic shift, etc.*
  - CMP
    - *Look for electrolyte abnormalities (hyponatremia), glucose, elevated LFTs, etc.*
  - PT/PTT/INR
    - *Look for bleeding abnormalities*

Imaging:

- Head CT or MRI (preferred)
  - Can do after LP if immunocompetent with no hx of recent head trauma, normal mental status, no papilledema or focal neuro defects, age <60, no seizure, no known CNS cancer, and no sinusitis
  - Otherwise, do LP after head CT or MRI
- Other imaging if warranted (CXR)

Diagnostic Workup and CSF Analysis of Suspected CNS Infection:

FAILS workup:

- If have any of FAILS → give dexamethasone, then, antibiotics, get CT, then do lumbar puncture
- If don't have any of FAILS → get lumbar puncture, then give dexamethasone then antibiotics (don't need a CT)
- **FAILS:**
    - Focal neurological deficit
    - Altered mental status, or **A**ge >60
    - **I**mmunosuppressed
    - **L**esion over the site of lumbar puncture
    - **S**eizure

LP studies:

- **Initial LP studies to order:**
    - Mostly depends on the clinical context
    - **Always order** opening pressure, WBC count, RBC count, glucose, CSF/serum glucose, protein, gram stain, culture
    - Can order PCR for enterovirus, HSV, ZVZ
    - Can order serology for HIV, enterovirus, and arthropod borne viruses
    - Can order CSF cryptococcal Ag, fungal culture
    - VDRL for syphilis
    - CXF AFB stain and TB PCR, TB culture

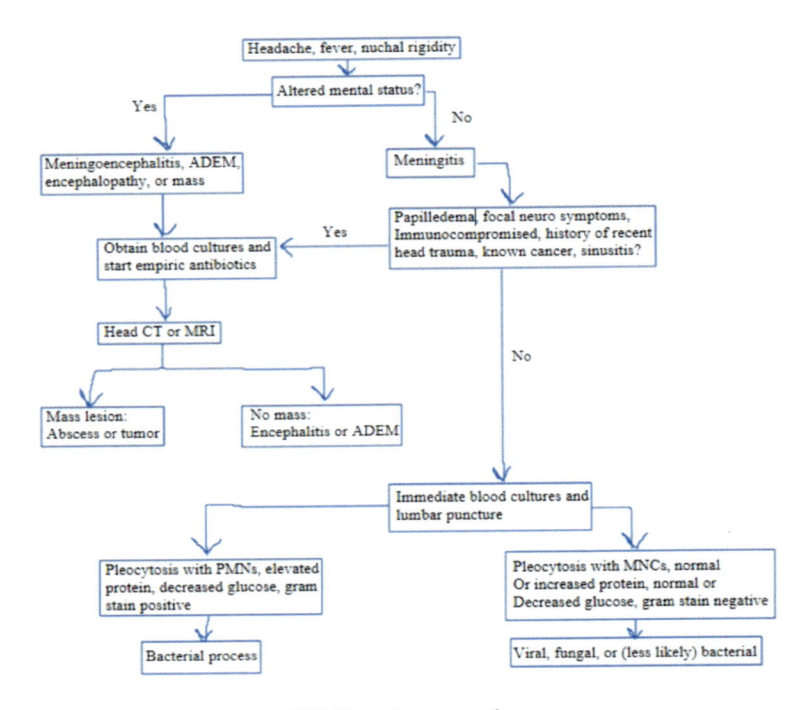

```
Headache, fever, nuchal rigidity
         │
   Altered mental status?
   ┌─────┴─────┐
  Yes          No
   │            │
Meningoencephalitis, ADEM,   Meningitis
encephalopathy, or mass         │
                    Papilledema, focal neuro symptoms,
         ┌──Yes────Immunocompromised, history of recent
         │         head trauma, known cancer, sinusitis?
Obtain blood cultures and
start empiric antibiotics             │
         │                            No
   Head CT or MRI                     │
   ┌─────┴─────┐                      │
Mass lesion:   No mass:               │
Abscess or     Encephalitis           │
tumor          or ADEM                │
                              Immediate blood cultures and
                              lumbar puncture
                         ┌────────────┴────────────┐
              Pleocytosis with PMNs,      Pleocytosis with MNCs, normal
              elevated protein,           Or increased protein, normal or
              decreased glucose,          Decreased glucose, gram stain negative
              gram stain positive
                    │                              │
             Bacterial process       Viral, fungal, or (less likely) bacterial
```

CSF Study Interpretation:

	Normal	**Bacterial**	**Viral**	**Fungal/TB**
Pressure	5-20	>30	Normal or mildly increased	
Appearance	Normal	Turbid	Clear	Fibrin web
Protein	0.18-0.45	>1	<1	0.1-0.5
Glucose	2.5-3.5	<2.2	Normal	1.6-2.5
Gram stain	Normal	60-90% positive	Normal	
Glucose-CSF:serum ratio	0.6	<0.4	>0.6	<0.4
White cell count	<3	>500	<1000	100-500
Other		90% PMNs	Monocytes ~10% have >90% PMNs ~30% have >50% PMNs	Monocytes

Treatment:

Empiric for bacterial meningitis:

- Start antibiotics within 60 minutes of patients arrival to the emergency room
- Start **dexamethasone** 10mg IV Q6h **before** first dose of antibiotics, for 4 days
    - **European Dexamethasone Study (2002, NEJM)**- Adjunctive therapy with dexamethasone reduces morbidity and mortality among patients with acute bacterial meningitis, particularly *Streptococcus pneumoniae* meningitis

Indication	Antibiotics
Preterm to infants <1 month old	Ampicillin + cefotaxime
1-3 months old	Ampicillin + cefotaxime or ceftriaxone
Immunocompetent >3 months- <55 years old	**Ceftriaxone + vancomycin**
Adults >55 or any age with alcoholism or other debilitating illness	**Ampicillin** + ceftriaxone or cefotaxime + vancomycin
Hospital acquired meningitis, post-neurosurgery, neutropenic, or impaired cell-mediated immunity	Ampicillin + ceftazidime or meropenem + vancomycin

- Acyclovir if considering HSV encephalitis
- **Tailor specific therapy once culture susceptibilities come back**
- If meningococcal meningitis, Rifampin 600mg PO BID x 2 days for close contacts
- **Essentials:**
    - **Dexamethasone before antibiotics**
    - **Ceftriaxone and vancomycin for all adults**
    - **Add ampicillin if also immunocompromised**

Viral and aseptic meningitis treatment:

- Mostly symptomatic treatment with analgesics, antipyretics, and anti-emetics
- Acyclovir PO or IV if caused by HSV 1 or 2 or severe EBV/VZV
- Seriously ill patients:
    - Acyclovir IV
    - Followed by acyclovir PO 5 times/day or famciclovir PO TID or valacyclovir TID for 7-14 days
    - If LP is negative for HSV encephalitis, but still have a high clinical suspicion for HSV, continue acyclovir, **and repeat LP 3-7 days after first LP for HSV PCR**
- HIV:
    - Start HAART
    - Vaccination for MMR, varivax, and zostavax for prevention
- If suspect TB:
    - Dexamethasone + RIPE therapy
- If suspect fungal:
    - Amphotericin B liposomal + 5-FU

Etiology:

- Bacterial:
    - **Strep pneumoniae** (30-60%)
        - Osler's triad- Meningitis + pneumonia + endocarditis
    - **N. meningitidis** (10-35%)
        - Rash, <30 years old
        - Complement C5-9 deficiency, vaccine (not type B)
    - H. influenza (<5%)
        - Decreased incidence due to the vaccine
        - Look for CSF leak, recent neurosurgery, trauma, mastoiditis
    - Listeria monocytogenes (5-10%)
        - Neonates, pregnant women, >60, alcoholics, immunosuppressed
        - Dairy and raw meat
    - Staph (5%)
        - CSF shunt (epidermidis) or following neurosurgery or head trauma (aureus)
    - Group B streptococci
        - Infants
            - S. agalactiae too
    - Gram negative rods
- Aseptic:
    - Viral:
        - Enterovirus (most common cause)
        - HIV
        - HSV (2 > 1)
        - VZV
        - Mumps
        - Lymphatic choriomeningitis virus
        - Adenovirus
        - Polio
        - CMV
        - EBV
        - West nile virus
        - Arbovirus
    - Parameningeal focus of infection:
        - Brain abscess
        - Epidural abscess
        - Septic thrombophlebitis
        - Subdural empyema
    - TB, fungal, spirochetal:
        - Lyme disease
        - Syphilis
        - Cryptococcus
        - Leptospirosis
        - RMSF
        - Coxiella
        - Ehrlichia
    - Medications:
        - TMP/SMX
        - NSAIDs
        - IVIG and antilymphocyte IG

- Penicillin
- Isoniazid
- Lamotrignine
  - Systemic illness:
    - SLE
    - Sarcoidosis
    - Behcet's syndrome
    - Sjogrens
    - Rheumatoid arthritis
  - Neoplasm:
    - Intracranial tumor (or cyst)
    - Lymphoma
  - Partially treated bacterial meningitis

Risk Factors:

- Sinusitis
- Otitis media
- Alcohol
- Diabetes
- Splenectomy
- Complement deficiency
- Head trauma
- Neurosurgery
- Unvaccinated
- Military barracks
- College dormitories
- Elderly
- HIV
- Immunocompromised
- Geography
- STD's
- Pregnancy

Pathogenesis:

- S. Pneumoniae/N. meningiditis colonize the nasopharynx by attaching to epithelial cells and are transported across membrane via vacuoles or through tight junctions to get to the blood stream
- Avoid phagocytosis due to polysaccharide capsule, reach the choroid plexus and go to the CSF
- Multiply rapidly in the CSF due to absence of effective host immune defenses (few WBCs and few complement/Ig's) → decreased opsonization
- **Critical event → inflammatory reaction induced by invading pathogen → immune response causes the neurologic sequalae** (NOT the organism)
- Bacteria lysed → release of cell wall components (LPS, teichoic acid, peptidoglycans), which induces **meningeal irritation from inflammatory cytokines and chemokines**
- TNF-alpha, interleukin 1beta released
- Cytokine response increases CSF proteins and leukocytosis
- Excitatory amino acids, ROS → cell death of brain cells

- TNF alpha and IL-1beta increase the vascular permeability which causes **vasogenic edema and leakage of serum proteins into the CSF, which obstructs CSF → hydrocephalus (herniation) and interstitial edema**
- Cytokines upregulate selectins → leukocyte migration into the CSF
- Neutrophil degranulation → toxin metabolites that cause edema, cell injury, and death
- Initially get increased cerebral blood flow, soon after get decreased blood flow from autoregulation

Complications:

- Recurrence
- Death
- Coma
- Cerebral edema
- Permanent neurologic sequelae
- **Cushing reflex**:
    - Bradycardia
    - HTN
    - Irregular respirations
- **Hearing loss**
- Memory loss
- Learning disabilities
- Seizures
- Subdural empyema
- Shock

Admission Orders:

- Admit to ICU
- Diagnosis meningitis
- Condition guarded
- Vital signs Q4h with neuro checks Q2h x 24h
- Allergies
- Activity Bed rest for first 24h, then ad lib
- Nursing droplet precautions, fall precautions, call for temp > 38.5C, HR > 110, systolic BP <100, or changing neurologic status
- Diet NPO for now, assess ability to swallow safely next day
- Fluids sepsis fluid resuscitation
- Meds:
    - Dexamethasone 10mg IV Q6h x 4 days before antibiotics
    - See antibiotic therapy above
- Labs/diagnostics:
    - Blood cultures x 2 before antibiotics
    - CT of brain
    - LP with CSF for cell count, differential, gram stain, culture, protein, glucose, PCR of suspected organisms if needed
    - CBC with diff
    - CMP
    - PT/PTT/INR

Discharge Information:

- Typically requires 2 + weeks of antibiotics parenterally
- At least 6 days in the hospital
- Outpatient if afebrile, stable, and no neurologic abnormalities
- Safe home environment
- PICC line
- Follow up with infectious disease or neurologist in 1 week

Additional Notes:

- Important clinical trials:
    - **European Dexamethasone Study (2002, NEJM)-** Adjunctive therapy with dexamethasone reduces morbidity and mortality among patients with acute bacterial meningitis, particularly *Streptococcus pneumoniae* meningitis

Cellulitis

Definitions:

Cellulitis- inflammation of the subcutaneous connective tissue

History:

The classic symptoms of cellulitis are explained by rubor, tumor, calor, dolor. That is, redness, swelling, heat, and pain. If you see symptoms of cellulitis, it is important to ask questions about how this infection was acquired. Signs of sepsis should be sought.

CC:

HPI:

- COLIDDERRS
    - *A patient with an ulcer, puncture, laceration, that has a rash that is warm, hot, tender, which has clear demarcations*
- Spreading?
    - *Where did it start?*
    - *How fast has it spread?*
- Fever/chills?
    - *Signs of infection*
- N/V?
    - *If they can't tolerate PO medications they will need admitted*
- Bites?
    - *What kind of animal?*
    - *Can change the choice of antibiotic*
- Catheters?
    - *How long has it been in?*
    - *Any purulent material coming out?*
- Puncture?
    - *What made the puncture?*
- Draining?
    - *Describe the draining material*
    - *When did it start, and has it changed?*
- Hot-tub use?
    - *Can lead to hot tub folliculitis, especially if diabetic, caused by pseudomonas*
- Salt or fresh water exposure?
    - *Can get infections by specific bugs, like Erysipelothrix (fish, swine), M. marinum (fish), vibrio vulnificus in cirrhotics*
- Gardening?
    - *Sporothrix if exposed to rose thorns*
- Fish/oyster exposure?
    - *See above*
- Numbness?
    - *Can have numbness in certain infections, like necrotizing fasciitis*

ROS:

PMH:

- Hx of MRSA?
    - *Can make you more susceptible to MRSA infection again as the person may be a host now*
- Hx of PVD?
    - *Can look like cellulitis, but also makes them more susceptible to infections as immune cells can't get to tissues as well*
- Hx of Venous stasis?
    - *Can look like cellulitis if develop venous stasis ulcers, but also makes them more susceptible to infections*
- Hx of CHF?
    - *Can lead to venous stasis ulcers that looks like infections*
- Hx of Diabetes?
    - *Can make you more susceptible to pseudomonas infections, and osteomyelitis, and to neuropathy where they can't feel a wound*

Surgical H:

Social H:

- Alcohol, smoking, recreational drugs, job, living situation, sexual history

Family H:

Allergies:

Medications:

Physical Examination:

Vital signs, mental status, and toxicity of the patient are the most important. Also, if there is a wound, examining it for pus and if bone is visible is very important.

- Vital signs
    - Fever, tachycardia, hypotension, signs of sepsis
- Mental status exam
    - Altered mental status may show signs of systemic infection
- Purulent drainage or exudate?
    - More likely a sign of staph infection where MRSA coverage should be initiated empirically
- Abscess?
    - Sign of infection that needs to be drained
- Carbuncle?
    - Sign of infection that needs to be drained/treated
- Spreading?
    - ED will usually mark the margins, spreading makes it more serious
- Puncture marks?
    - Can change the type of antibiotic chosen, especially if what type of animal that bit them is known

- Heat?
  - Sign of infection
- Check pulses
  - Need to make sure pulses are present, as absence may make antibiotics ineffective and may need surgical treatment

Labs:

- Blood cultures x 2
- CBC with diff
  - Leukocytosis, anemia, neutrophilic shift, etc.
- CMP
  - Electrolyte abnormalities, glucose, LFTs, BUN/Cr
- If open or abscess, drain and culture
- ESR and CRP to help rule out osteomyelitis if indicated

Imaging:

- X-ray, then MRI if suspecting osteomyelitis
  - X-ray to rule out other disease with X-ray (like gas gangrene, necrotizing fasciitis, osteomyelitis)

Admission:

- Admit if any of the following are present:
  - Signs of systemic toxicity or concern for rapidly spreading infection
  - Patient is unable to keep affected leg elevated (if leg infection)
  - Pt is unable to tolerate PO antibiotics

Treatment:

- **Empiric treatment:**
  - Purulent:
    - Need to cover MRSA empirically at first, tailor afterwards
    - Clindamycin, Bactrim, doxycycline, linezolid (all oral meds)
    - Vancomycin or linezolid if purulence with extensive disease or signs of systemic toxicity
  - Non-purulent:
    - Less likely MRSA or staph, more likely strep
    - Cephalexin, dicloxacillin, clindamycin (all oral meds)
  - Animal/Human bite:
    - Augmentin 875/125 mg PO BID if prophylactic
    - Unasyn 1.5-3g IV Q6h if established infection
    - All human bites require augmentin, animal bites only require it if looks like extensive infection
  - Cellulitis IV (staph or strep):
    - Nafcillin or oxacillin
  - MRSA IV:
    - Vancomycin 1g IV Q 12h
  - Necrotizing fasciitis:

- Rapid spread through fascial planes, strep pneumo, rapidly expanding cellulitis, **pain out of proportion to exam, numbness of the area**, diabetics, blue-grey discoloration to skin, use LRINEC score
          - Clindamycin + imipenem (or zosyn) + vancomycin and **debridement**
        - Gas gangrene:
          - Dirty wound, gas producing organisms (clostridium perfringens, bacteroides fragilis, strep pyogenes), cellulitis with **crepitus**
          - Clindamycin 600-900 mg IV Q6-8h + Penicillin G 4 million units IV Q 4h
- **Outpatient cellulitis empiric:**
    - Cephalexin, augmentin, clindamycin
    - If MRSA is suspected, Bactrim, clindamycin, or doxycycline + amoxicillin or linezolid
- Ancillary treatment:
    - Leg elevation
    - Wound dressing/cleaning

Etiology:

- **Big question is staph or not staph**
- **Streptococcus**
- **Staphylococcus**
- MRSA
- Strep pyogenes
- Pasteurella (cat/dog bite)
- Eikenella (bites)
- Fusobacterium
- Bacteroides
- Aeromonas (lakes)
- Pseudomonas (hot tub, diabetes, penetrating wound)
- Erysipelothrix (fish, swine)
- M. marinum (fish)
- Vibrio vulnificus (fish in a cirrhotic patient)
- M. fortuitum (footbaths/pedicures, recent shaving)

Additional Notes:

-

Osteomyelitis

Definitions:

Osteomyelitis- infection of bone due to hematogenous or direct spread from a contiguous source

History:

With someone who has suspected osteomyelitis, it is important to assess for toxicity of the patient, and to inquire about risk factors that can lead to osteomyelitis.

CC:

HPI:

- COLIDDERRS
    - *Patient with bone pain and cellulitis that you can probe down to the bone*
- F/C?
    - *Common symptoms of osteomyelitis*
- Drainage?
    - *Describe it*
    - *Has it changed or gotten worse?*
- Pain?
    - *Where and how severe?*
- Trauma to the area?
    - *What was done?*
    - *Was it a penetrating wound?*

ROS:

PMH:

- Hx of Diabetes?
    - *More susceptible to osteomyelitis, and to pseudomonas infection, and to neuropathy*
- Hx of Neuropathy?
    - *Can make them not feel ulcers on their feet, wounds, etc. that can lead to osteomyelitis that is not even felt*
- Hx of TB?
    - *History of TB can lead to disseminated secondary TB which can become osteomyelitis*

Surgical H:

- Recent surgery?
    - *More susceptible to infections at the incision site that can lead to osteomyelitis*
- Prosthetic joints?

- More susceptible to certain types of osteomyelitis (70% is due to staph (aureus and coagulase negative), 10% strep, 10% gram negative rods, P. acnes)

Social H:

- Alcohol, smoking, recreational drugs, job, living situation, sexual history

Family H:

Allergies:

Medications:

Physical Examination:

The general appearance of the patient to assess for toxicity is important. A thorough exam of the wound is necessary, as it is important to know if the bone is exposed.

- Vital signs
  - Fever, tachycardia, tachypnea, SaO2, signs of SIRS/sepsis
- Check for systemic symptoms
- Check for drainage
- Abscess?
- Fluctuance?
- Bone exposed?

Differential Diagnosis:

- Cellulitis
  - *Fever, well demarcated margins, erythema, but no deep wound infection*
- Septic arthritis
  - *Have other symptoms of the potential source, like endocarditis symptoms*
- Gout
  - *Very erythematous, usually at MTP joint but can be elsewhere, usually no penetrating wound, no X-ray or MRI findings, can be after alcohol binge or red meat consumption or during acute illness*
- Diabetic or arterial insufficiency
  - *Usually no penetrating wound, no fever*
- TB or mycotic bone infection
  - *Have had a history of TB or mycosis infection*
- Rheumatic fever
  - *Sore throat, polyarthritis, carditis, syndenham chorea, erythema marginatum, subcutaneous nodules, usually no penetrating wound*
- Metastatic cancer
  - *Can spread to bone and mimic osteomyelitis*
- Multiple myeloma
  - *Can have back pain mimicking vertebral osteomyelitis, but will have hypercalcemia, renal failure, anemia, and punched out lytic lesions*
- Ewings sarcoma

- o   *Younger child with bone pain*
- Avascular necrosis
  - o   *Bone pain very severe, can have risk factors avascular necrosis (such as sickle cell)*
- Pyelonephritis
  - o   *Can mimic vertebral osteomyelitis, will have abnormal UA, no penetrating wounds*
- Pancreatitis
  - o   *Can mimic vertebral osteomyelitis, will have typical symptoms of pancreatitis (epigastric pain radiating to back, elevated amylase and lipase, etc.)*
- Charcots foot
  - o   *Unilateral swelling with increase in temperature, erythema, joint effusion, bone resorption, with intact skin and loss of sensation of the area, no fever, pain is less than suspected*
- Fracture
  - o   *Trauma and X-ray evidence of fracture with no infectious signs/symptoms*

Labs:

- Blood cultures x 2
- Bone swab/biopsy (NOT wound swab)
- CBC with diff
  - o   Leukocytosis, anemia, thrombocytopenia, neutrophilic shift, etc.
- ESR
  - o   Usually do not trend this, as it is a marker for more prolonged inflammation as opposed to CRP
- CRP
  - o   Trend this throughout their stay, more used as a marker of if they are getting better with treatment rather than to diagnose it at the beginning
- CMP
  - o   Electrolyte abnormalities, glucose, LFTs, BUN/Cr
- UA with culture

Imaging:

- Plain radiographs 1st if no neurologic symptoms
- MRI- gold standard, do quickly if neuro symptoms are present
- CT- less specific than MRI, can guide biopsy of the bone
- PET scan for patients with implants and for patients in whom several foci are suspected
- Ankle-brachial index if foot, to know if ortho or vascular surgery sees patient

Etiologies and Treatment:

- <u>General treatment:</u>
  - o   Surgical debridement needed for most cases
  - o   If not toxic, do not give any antibiotics at first
  - o   If toxic, do give empiric antibiotics
- <u>Foot osteomyelitis:</u>

- Diabetic, arterial insufficiency, neuropathy
- S. aureus 40-50%, anaerobes 20-35%, gram negative rods 20-30%
- Treatment:
  - Wound debridement + ~6 weeks of antibiotics
  - Vancomycin for MRSA coverage plus
  - Zosyn or cefepime if concerned for pseudomonas
  - If not concerned for pseudomonas, can do ceftriaxone and metronidazole

- Vertebral osteomyelitis:
  - Fever, radiculopathy, weakness, bowel/bladder incontinence, paralysis
  - Acute- staph aureus 40-50%, strep 12%, gram negative rods 20%, E. coli 9%, Pseudomonas 6%
  - Subacute/chronic- TB, Brucella, Strep viridians (if endocarditis present), Candida (IV drug abuse)
  - Treatment:
    - If no sepsis, don't give antibiotics until the organism is identified (may need to do CT guided biopsy of vertebra)
    - IV antibiotics for ~6 weeks
    - Vancomycin + cefepime (or zosyn)
    - Surgical debridement if implant present, or necrotic bone is present

- Osteomyelitis in long bones:
  - Pain, low grade fever, erythema, swelling, pus discharge
  - Etiologies same as vertebral osteomyelitis
  - Treatment:
    - Acute hematogenous → 4-6 weeks of IV antibiotics
    - Recurrence → debridement with long term antibiotics
    - Implant → fluoroquinolone + rifampin, possible removal of implant

- Periprosthetic joint infection:
  - Acute- pain of new onset
  - Chronic- joint effusion, pain, implant loosening, sinus tract formation present
  - 70% is due to staph (aureus and coagulase negative), 10% strep, 10% gram negative rods, P. acnes
  - Treatment:
    - Ortho + infectious disease + plastics + microbiologist multidisciplinary team at a specialized surgery center
    - Surgery + rifampin + a fluoroquinolone long term

- Sternal osteomyelitis:
  - Occurs after sternal surgery
  - S. aureus 40-50%, coagulase negative staph 30%, enterococci 5-12%, Gram negative rods 15-25%, pseudomonas with IV drug abuse
  - Treatment:
    - Antibiotics with beta-lactam + vancomycin, linezolid, or daptomycin if MRSA is suspected
    - Rifampin
    - Possible surgery

Risk Factors:

- Recent surgery

- Implants
- Trauma
- IV drug abuse
- Diabetes
- Catheters
- Immunosuppressed

Complications:

- Persistent pain
- New onset neuro impairments
- Abscesses
- Persistence of infection
- Sinus tract formation
- Amputation

Admission Orders:

- Admit to floor
- Diagnosis osteomyelitis
- Condition stable
- Vital signs routine
- Allergies
- Activity up as tolerated, with assistance
- Nursing routine. Call for temp > 38.5C, systolic BP <100, HR >110
- Diet regular
- Fluids sepsis resuscitation
- Meds:
    - Acetaminophen 650mg PO Q6h prn pain/fever
    - Antibiotics as above
    - Heparin 5000 U SubQ Q8h or lovenox
- Labs/diagnostics:
    - CBC with diff
    - ESR
    - CRP
    - CMP
    - Blood cultures x 2
    - UA with culture
    - Plain X-ray
    - MRI

Discharge Information:

- Prolonged IV antibiotic planning
- Vertebral osteomyelitis → 4-6 weeks of IV antibiotics
- PICC line
- Follow up with labs and imaging

Additional Notes:

-

Miscellaneous Topics in Internal Medicine

Inpatient Diabetes Management

Approach:

- **Stop all oral diabetes medications**
- Use both long acting (basal) and short acting (prandial) insulin
    - Long acting:
        - Lantus
        - Levemir
    - Short acting:
        - Novolog
        - Humalog
- Figure out the **total daily insulin (TDI):**
    - If Cr <1.5, age <70, and blood glucose >180:
        - Use **0.5 U/kg**
    - If Cr >1.5, or age >70, or blood glucose <180:
        - Use **0.3 U/kg**
- **½ of the TDI is given in long acting form QHS or QAM**
- **½ of the TDI is given in short acting form between meals three times a day**
- **Add sliding scale insulin** (SSI) on top of what was calculated
    - Make sure the SSI is the same type of insulin you are giving as the short acting form
- Each new day, look at the SSI given the day before, and add that amount to the old TDI to get your **new TDI**
- Can either add 20% of the total daily insulin and divide that equally into long acting and short acting, or use new TDI and divide that into long and short acting
- **Example patient:**
    - A 55 year old male is admitted for pneumonia. He is on two oral medications at home for diabetes. His Cr is 1.0, and his blood glucose is 200. He weighs 100 kg
        - He meets criteria to do **0.5 U/kg** for the TDI
        - TDI= 100 X 0.5= 50 units of insulin total
        - Long acting insulin = ½ TDI = 50 X 0.5 = **25 Units of Lantus or Levemir**
        - Short acting insulin = ½ TDI = 50 X 0.5 = 25 Units of Novolog or Humalog
            - This gets divided between three meals
            - 25 U/3= **~8 U at each meal**
        - Add SSI
    - The next day you see he needed 2 units of Novolog between each meal for his SSI
        - This is 6 units more a day than scheduled
        - New TDI = old TDI + total SSI = 50 + 6 = 56
        - 56 X .20 = 11.2, add 5 to long acting, add 6 total to short acting (long 30 and short 31 or 10 with meals)
        - Or divide 56 equally into long vs short, so 28 long, and 27 short (9 each meal)

Hemoptysis

Differential:

- **Pneumonia**
- **Bronchitis**
- Bronchiectasis
- Aspergillus
- Autoimmune
- TB
- Tumor
- Lung abscess
- Embolism (air, placenta, DVT/PE, fat/cholesterol)
- Cystic fibrosis
- Coagulopathy
- AVM
- Mitral valve

Things to Consider:

- Have to separate hemoptysis from hematemesis
- **Ask the patient directly if it is blood with cough, or blood with vomit**
- Look in the mouth and nose for oropharyngeal trauma
- **Consults:**
    - Pulmonology if in lung (hemoptysis)
    - GI if in GI system (hematemesis)
    - ENT if in oropharynx (oral nasal trauma)

Back Pain

- **Admit** patient if they have any **red flags:**
    - Focal neurologic deficit (loss of bowel/bladder function, weakness, loss of motor or sensation)
    - Fever (infectious)
    - Percussive tenderness (fracture)
    - History of cancer (mets)
    - Coagulopathy (hematoma)
    - Immunosuppressed (infection)
    - Spinal procedure recently (abscess, hematoma)
- If they have red flags, best imaging modality is **MRI**
- **Differential:**
    - Visceral (pancreas, aorta, hematoma, kidneys, uterus)
    - Spine (fracture, abscess, osteomyelitis, Pott's, metastasis)
    - Nerves (herniation, osteophytes, spinal stenosis, cauda equina, spondylolisthesis)
    - Musculoskeletal (strain, sprain, overuse)
    - Autoimmune (ankylosing spondylitis, RA, other seronegatives)

Diarrhea

- **Admit** the patient if:
  - Dehydration
  - Travel recently
  - On antibiotics
  - Blood in diarrhea
  - Duration > 5 days

Differential/Approach:

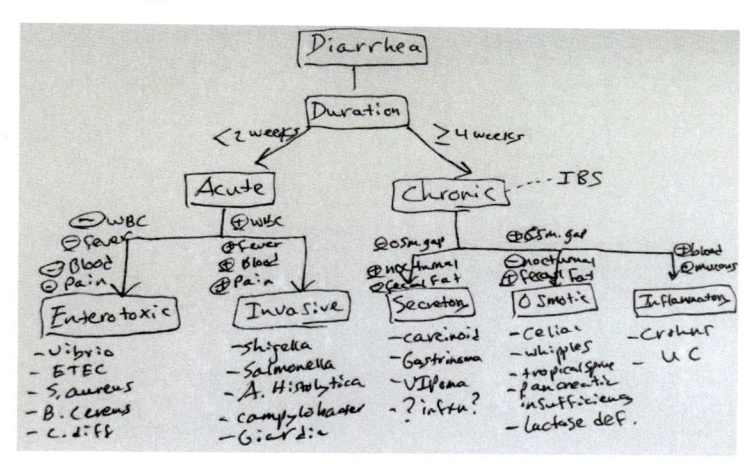

[Flowchart: Diarrhea → Duration → <2 weeks (Acute) or ≥4 weeks (Chronic ··· IBS)

Acute:
- ⊖WBC, ⊖fever, ⊖blood, ⊖pain → **Enterotoxic**: Vibrio, ETEC, S. aureus, B. cereus, C. diff
- ⊕WBC, ⊕fever, ⊕blood, ⊕pain → **Invasive**: Shigella, Salmonella, A. histolytica, Campylobacter, Giardia

Chronic:
- ≥Osm gap, ⊕nocturnal, ⊖fecal fat → **Secretory**: carcinoid, Gastrinoma, VIPoma, ? inftn?
- ⊕Osm gap, ⊖nocturnal, ⊕fecal fat → **Osmotic**: celiac, whipples, tropical sprue, pancreatic insufficiency, lactase def.
- ⊕blood, ⊕mucous → **Inflammatory**: Crohns, UC]

Management:

- If have **NO warning signs** (fever, significant abdominal pain, blood or pus in stools, >6 stools/day, severe dehydration, immunosuppression, elderly, duration >7 days, or hospital acquired) **and can tolerate PO**:
  - Supportive treatment only
  - Oral hydration, loperamide, bismuth
- If moderate dehydration:
  - 50-200 mL/kg/day of oral solution (1/2 tsp baking soda, 8 tsp sugar, and 8 ounces OJ diluted to 1 L with water) or Gatorade, etc.
- If severe dehydration:
  - Lactated ringers or NS
- For travelers diarrhea:
  - Bismuth or rifaximin for prophylaxis and empiric treatment
- Empiric antibiotics for non-hospital acquired inflammatory diarrhea:
  - A **fluoroquinolone** (such as ciprofloxacin, levofloxacin, ofloxacin) X 5-7 days
- If **C. diff:**
  - Contact precautions if even suspect C. diff
  - Depends how sick they are
  - Metronidazole PO for first time or first recurrence and moderate illness

o If severe or 2nd recurrence, vancomycin PO

Alcohol Withdrawal

Clinical Features:

- Minor withdrawal symptoms- **6-48h after last drink**: mild anxiety, tremulousness, headache, tachycardia, fever, insomnia, n/v
- Mostly applicable to long term users who stop abruptly, not binge drinkers
- **Withdrawal seizures**- typically **within 48h after last drink**: if untreated **1/3 goes to delirium tremens**, which can be life threatening
    - Delirium tremens is disorientation, agitation, hallucinations, tachycardia, hypertension, fever, diaphoresis, seizures possibly
    - Begins 48-96 hours after last drink
    - Lasts 5-7 days
- Differential:
    - CNS infection or bleed
    - Seizure
    - Drug overdose
    - Acute liver failure
    - GI bleed

Clinical Institute Withdrawal Assessment Scale (CIWA):

- 10 criteria categories, each category is scored from 0-7 except orientation which is 0-4
- Total score <8 is none to mild withdrawal
- Total score 8-15 is mild withdrawal
- Total score 26-20 is moderate withdrawal
- Total score >20 is severe withdrawal
- Consider transfer to ICU if score >35
- Categories:
    - N/v
    - Tremor
    - Paroxysmal sweats
    - Anxiety
    - Agitation
    - Tactile disturbances (itching, numbness, hallucinations)
    - Auditory disturbances
    - Visual disturbances
    - Headache/fullness in head
    - Orientation/clouding of sensorium

Treatment:

- Thiamine if NPO 'banana bag', NS 100mg thiamine, 1g folate, then glucose to prevent Wernicke's encephalopathy
- Multivitamin PO if can tolerate
- Vitals Q4h if CIWA <10, otherwise Q1h
- Cardiac monitoring, continuous pulse ox, fall/seizure/aspiration precautions, social work referral, dietitian referral

- **Benzodiazepines:**
    - Chlordiazepoxide (Librium) (long acting), if PO
    - Lorazepam (short acting), if NPO 2mg IV Q2h for CIWA <10, Q1h if CIWA 10-15, 4mg Q1h for CIWA >15
    - Diazepam (long acting) can be used instead of lorazepam
    - **Use a long acting with a short acting prn**
    - Can use oxazepam or lorazepam if cirrhosis
    - Regimen- diazepam 10-15 mg IV Q10-15 min or lorazepam 2-4 mg IV Q15-20 min until appropriate sedation achieved, then titrate to CIWA-Ar scale
- If refractory to benzodiazepines, consider benzo gtt, phenopbarbital, or propofol (& intubation)
- **Prophylaxis:**
    - If minimal symptoms or asymptomatic (CIWA <8) but prolonged heavy alcohol use or history of withdrawal seizures or DTs
    - Librium 25-100 mg (based on severity of alcohol use) Q6h x 24h, then 25-50 mg Q6h x 2 days
- Replace Mg, P, and K, fluids

Approach to LFTs

Markers:

- **Markers of liver function (hepatocellular function):**
    - **Chronic markers:**
        - Total protein
        - Albumin
        - INR
    - **Acute markers:**
        - AST
        - ALT
- **Markers of biliary function:**
    - Direct bilirubin
    - Alkaline phosphatase
- **Makers of hemolysis:**
    - Total bilirubin, direct and indirect

Meaning of Markers:

- **Hemolysis:**
    - If total bilirubin is elevated, with mostly indirect bilirubin, then it's a sign of hemolysis
- **Obstructive or post-hepatic pathologies:**
    - Elevated direct bilirubin and alkaline phosphatase
        - Alkaline phosphatase comes from both biliary tree and bone, so an elevated alkaline phosphatase can be confirmed to be from the biliary tree by ordering a **GGT**, which only comes from bone
- **Chronic hepatocellular disease:**
    - Decreased total protein, decreased albumin, increased INR
- **Acute hepatocellular disease:**
    - Elevated AST and ALT

- o If AST:ALT > 2:1 ratio, then most likely from alcoholic hepatitis and cirrhosis
- o AST elevations alone can come from muscle, can show elevated CK levels too (ie rhabdo)
- o **AST/ALT in the 1,000's**
    - Shock liver, acute viral hepatitis (A, B), autoimmune hepatitis, acetaminophen poisoning, aflatoxin, Budd Chiari

- **Protein gap:**
    - o Difference between the total protein and albumin
    - o If it's >4, you have immunoglobulins
        - Think HIV, Hep C, and multiple myeloma
- **Low albumin:**
    - o Loses it in urine (nephrosis, nephrotic syndrome)
    - o Can't build it (cirrhosis)
    - o Can't absorb it (gastrosis, protein malnutrition)

Approach to Pain Control

- Pain is often undertreated in the hospital
- Complete absence of pain is often an unrealistic goal
- Patients should be frequently reassessed during analgesic treatment
- Scheduled analgesics are better than prn administration
- Before prescribing pain meds, always consider comorbidities, allergies, drug interactions, and potential side effects
- **Select alternative agents to meperidine and codeine** to limit side effects and drug interactions
- Questions to ask yourself:
    - o Does the patient only ask for pain medications when you are in the room?
    - o Do others observe different behaviors when you leave the room?
    - o Is the patient 'splitting' the staff, playing one against the other?
    - o Is the patient talking or resting comfortably?
        - This may be misleading in patients with chronic pain and should not be assumed to be a sign of deception in such patients
    - o Is the patient allergic to every pain medication except the one he or she is requesting?
    - o Is the patient unwilling to accept any adjunctive nonopioid treatment?
    - o Is the patient very sleepy or lethargic and still asking for more?
- **Equipotent analgesic doses of opioids:**
    - o Calculate the total opioid dose used in the previous 24 hours
    - o Convert the total dose to an oral morphine equivalent (use table below)
    - o Convert the oral morphine equivalent to the new opioid
    - o Give 50% of the calculated daily dose to account for incomplete cross-tolerance between opioids
    - o Schedule the dosing frequency based on the analgesic half life (ie for morphine Q4h, MS contin Q8-12h, oxycodone Q5h, Oxycontin Q12h)

- Divide the calculated 24 hour dosage by the number of doses to be given daily
- Add prn doses of the new opioid (short acting form) at 5% to 15% of the total daily dose for breakthrough pain

Drug	SQ/IV dose (mg)	PO dose (mg)	Duration (hours)	Half-life (hours)
Short half-life opioids				
Morphine	10	30	4	2-3.5
Hydrocodone	-	30	4	3-4
Oxycodone	-	20	4	3
Hydromorphone	1.5	7.5	4	2-3
Fentanyl	0.1	-	1-2	1.5-6
Long-acting opioids				
Methadone	-	1.7-6.7	4-48	15-60

Agent	Oral	Parenteral
Step 1: Mild pain- Nonopioid and/or adjuvant		
Acetaminophen	650 mg Q4h-6h prn or 1,000 mg Q6h prn (max: 4 g/d, 2 g/d if liver disease)	1,000 mg IV Q6h prn
Aspirin	325-650 mg Q4h-6h prn	-
Ibuprofen	200-800 mg Q6-8h prn	-
Ketorolac	10 mg Q4-6h prn (max: 40 mg/d)	30-60 mg IM or 15-30 mg IV X 1; 15-30 IM/IV Q6h prn
Gabapentin (for neuropathy)	Starting dose 300 mg QHS, titrating to a max of 3,600 mg/d divided Q8h	-
Pregabalin (for neuropathy)	100-600 mg/d, divided into 2-3 doses	-
Step 2: Moderate pain- opioid formulated for mild/moderate pain (and/or nonopioid, and/or adjuvant)		
Tramadol	25-100 mg Q4-6h (max: 400 mg/d)	-
Hydrocodone/acetaminophen (e.g. Vicodin, norco, lorcet)	5/325 mg tabs, 1-2 tabs Q4-6h prn	-
Oxycodone /acetaminophen (e.g. Percocet, tylox, roxicet)	5/325 mg tabs, 1-2 tabs Q4-6h prn	-
Step 3: Severe pain- opioid formulated for moderate/severe pain (and/or nonopioid, and/or adjuvant)		
Morphine	Immediate release tablets 10-30 mg Q2-4h prn Suppository 10-2- mg Q4h prn	2-10 SC/IM/IV Q2-6h prn
Morphine extended release (e.g. MS contin, oramorph SR)	15 mg Q8-12h	-
Hydromorphone (dilaudid)	2-4 mg Q3-4h prn	0.5-4 mg SC/IM/IV Q3-6h prn
Fentanyl	-	Transdermal 12/5-100 mcg/h IV 50-100 mcg Q1-2h

Approach to Reading Chest X-Rays

- **Be systematic so you don't miss anything**
- **Technique:**
    - Is the exposure correct?
        - Underexposure can cause you to see things that are not there
        - Overexposure can cause pathology to disappear
        - You should be able to faintly see the intervertebral disc spaces through the cardiac silhouette
    - Is the patient properly positioned?

- The spinous process and trachea should be midline, with clavicular heads equidistant from the spinous processes
  - Is it PA or AP?
    - PA and lateral views are best, only done if patient can stand
    - AP images are usually obtained emergently when patient can't stand
  - Was the image taken at full inspiration?
    - Small lung volumes can produce vascular crowding and apparent mediastinal widening and atelectasis
- **Lines and tubes:**
  - Check position of endotracheal tube if present (should be 2 cm above carina with 3-5 cm above being optimal)
  - Central venous catheters should follow expected venous courses, and generally terminate at the SVC near the level of the carina along the right aspect of the mediastinum
  - NG and enteric feeding tubes may be partially visualized, make sure they do not coil in esophagus or extend outward into the lung
- **Airway:**
  - Trachea should be midline and not deviated
    - If tension pneumothorax, trachea deviates away from lung pathology
    - In volume loss or lobar collapse, trachea deviates toward lung pathology
- **Bones:**
  - Look at the sternum, ribs, clavicles, spine, and shoulders for fractures, osteolytic or osteoblastic lesions, and arthritic changes
- **Diaphragm:**
  - Sides of diaphragm should be equal and slightly rounded, the right side may be higher
  - Elevation of one side may suggest paralysis, loss of lung volume on that side, diaphragmatic eventration, or diaphragmatic tear (in trauma)
  - Look for blunting of costophrenic angles for pleural effusions
  - Flat hemidiaphragms are indicative of hyperexpansion, often seen in COPD
  - Check for free air under the diaphragm on upright radiograph (bowel perforation)
- **Soft tissues:**
  - Examine the soft tissues for symmetry, subcutaneous air, edema, and breast tissue
- **Heart and mediastinum:**
  - Look at heart size, greater than half of the chest width suggests cardiomegaly or pericardial effusion
  - Aortic knob should be distinct
  - Mediastinal widening may indicate thoracic aortic dissection or aneurysm, left atrial dilation, mass, or mediastinal fat deposition in obese patients
  - Mediastinal deviation may be seen with tension pneumothorax
- **Hilar structures:**
  - Let hilum is usually 2-3 cm higher than the right
  - Enlarged hila suggests LAD or pulmonary artery enlargement
- **Lung markings:**

- Look for normal lung markings all the way out to the chest wall to rule out pneumothorax
    - If lung markings are not seen to the periphery, look for a thin white visceral pleural line (do not miss this)
- Normal lung markings taper as they travel out to the periphery and are smaller in the upper lungs
    - Lung markings in the upper lung fields that are as large or larger than those in the lower lung ("cephalization") suggests pulmonary edema
- Kerley's B lines (small linear densities perpendicular to the pleural surface often best seen in the lung bases) are seen in congestive heart failure
- Hyperlucent lungs with increased retrosternal clear space on the lateral image are seen in emphysema
- Examine the lungs for areas of consolidation and nodules
- Obscuration of all or part of the heart border (silhouette sign) implies that a lesion is contiguous with or abuts the heart border and likely lies within the right middle lobe or lingua
- A small pleural effusion is suggested by blunting of the costophrenic angle, best seen on the lateral image

Approach to Reading EKGs

Every EKG should be systematically read in the following order to not miss anything:

- Rate
- Rhythm
    - Pauses
    - Premature contractions
    - All P waves the same morphology in a single lead?
    - P before every QRS and vice versa
    - PR interval
    - QRS interval
- Axis
    - Look at leads I and AVF
- Hypertrophy
    - P wave morphology in V1 for atria
    - R/S in V1/2 and V5/6 for ventricles
- Infarction
    - Significant Q waves
    - ST changes
    - T wave inversion

Read a rhythm strip first, then look at 12 leads. **Every** patient of yours that gets an EKG should be read and interpreted by you. Always try to compare a previous EKG to a new one.

Rate:

- Count large boxes to get the following rate:
    - 300, 150, 100, 75, 60, 50, 40, etc.
- For bradycardia and irregular rhythms:

- Cycles/6 second strip X 10= rate
- 10 large boxes per cycle is a rate of 30 BPM

Rhythm:

- Identify basic rhythm, then scan for pauses, premature beats, irregularity, intervals, and abnormal waves
- P before every QRS
- QRS after every P
- PR interval
- QRS interval
- Has QRS vector shifted outside normal range?
    - See left axis deviation in left anterior hemiblock
    - See right axis deviation with left posterior hemiblock
- **Irregular rhythms:**
    - **Sinus arrhythmia-** physiological response to breathing; irregular rhythm that changes with inspiration/expiration (normal) 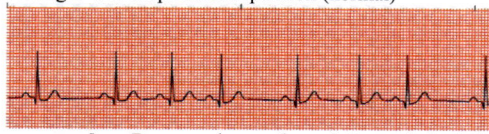
    - **Wandering pacemaker-** P waves change shape (≥3 morphologies) with a rate <**100 BPM**
    - **Multifocal atrial tachycardia-** P waves change shape (≥3 morphologies) with a rate of **>100 BPM** 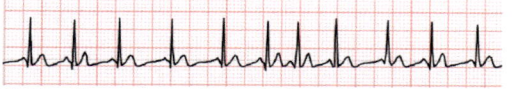
    - **Atrial fibrillation-** irregular ventricular rhythm with **no P waves** 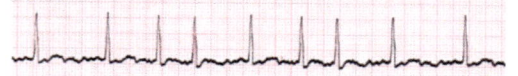
- **Escape beats:**
    - An unhealthy SA node may fail to emit a pacing stimulus (sinus block), producing a pause, that may produce an escape beat from a normally overdrive-suppressed automaticity focus
    - **Atrial escape beat-** a pause that produces a morphologically different P wave than the rest with a normal QRS interval 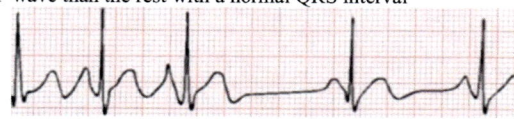
    - **Junctional escape beat-** a pause that produces no P wave with a normal QRS interval

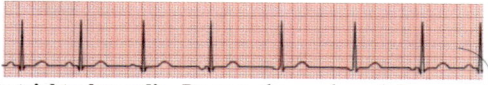

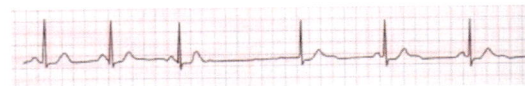

- **Ventricular escape beat-** a pause that produces no P wave with a widened QRS interval

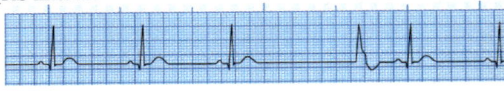

- **Escape rhythms:**
    - An unhealthy SA node may cease to produce a pacing stimulus (sinus arrest), causing a normally overdrive-suppressed automaticity focus to take over pacing responsibilities
    - The same as above, except instead of one beat occurring, it turns into the rhythm (multiple escape beats in a row)
- **Premature beats:**
    - An irritable automaticity focus may suddenly discharge, producing a premature beat
    - **Premature atrial complex (PAC)-** a premature beat with a morphologically different P wave than the rest with a normal QRS interval

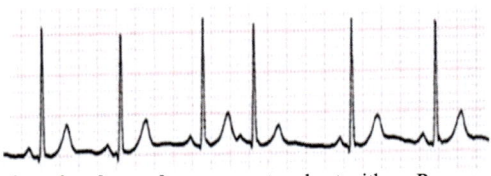

    - **Premature junctional complex-** a premature beat with no P wave and a normal QRS interval

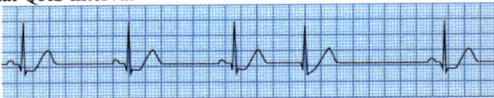

    - **Premature ventricular complex (PVC)-** a premature beat with no P wave and a widened QRS interval

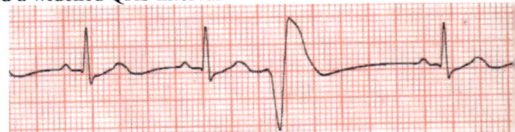

- **Tachyarrhythmias:**
    - Paroxysmal tachycardias (rate of 150-250, includes supraventricular tachycardias (paroxysmal atrial tachycardia (with and without block)) and paroxysmal junctional tachycardia), and paroxysmal ventricular tachycardia
    - Flutter rhythms have a rate of 250-350 BPM and include atrial flutter and ventricular flutter
    - Fibrillation rhythms have a rate of 350-450 BPM and include atrial fibrillation and ventricular fibrillation
    - **Paroxysmal atrial tachycardia-** an irritable focus discharging at 150-250 BPM with a visibly different P wave than before

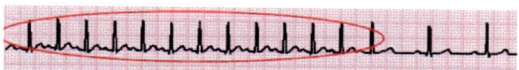

- o **Paroxysmal junctional tachycardia-** an AV junctional focus produces a rapid sequence of QRS-T cycles (no P waves) at 150-250 BPM (QRS interval may be slightly widened)

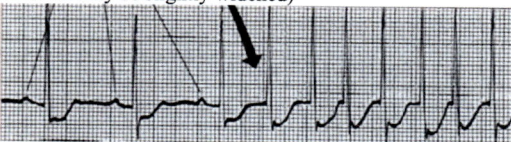

- o **Paroxysmal ventricular tachycardia-** a ventricular focus produces a rapid (150-250 BPM) sequence of PVC like wide ventricular complexes (QRS interval widened with no P waves)

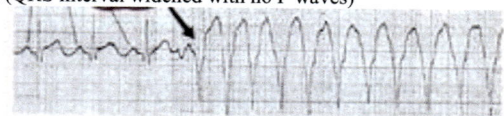

- o **Atrial flutter-** a continuous (sawtooth) rapid sequence of atrial complexes from a single rapid-firing atrial focus (**treatment**: CCB=BB, synchronized shock if unstable)

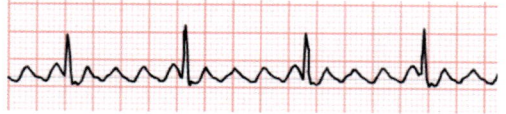

- o **Ventricular flutter-** a rapid series of smooth sine waves from a single rapid-firing ventricular focus, usually leading to ventricular fibrillation (also see Torsades de Pointes)(**treatment**: amiodarone, shock if unstable)

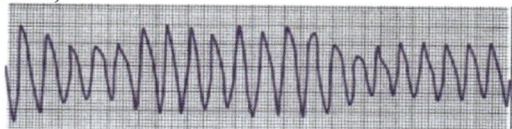

- o **Atrial fibrillation-** multiple atrial foci rapidly discharging produce a jagged baseline of tiny spikes, irregular ventricular rhythm with **no P waves** (**treatment**: CCB=BB, shock if unstable)

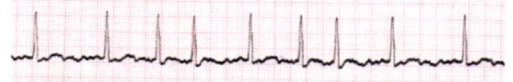

- o **Ventricular fibrillation-** multiple ventricular foci rapidly discharging produce a totally erratic ventricular rhythm without identifiable waves (**treatment**: amiodarone, unsynchronized shock if unstable)

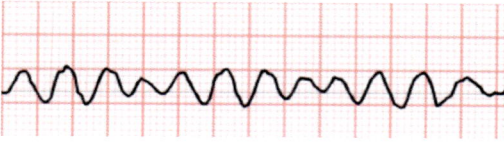

- **Blocks:**

- Scan PR interval to see if prolonged (>.2 secs), if they are getting longer, and if there are missed beats (AV blocks)
- Scan QRS interval to see if prolonged (>.12 secs) (bundle branch blocks)
- Look to see if QRS duration is normal or prolonged and an axis deviation is present (hemiblocks)
- **SA block-** an unhealthy SA node misses one or more cycles (sinus pause), an escape beat may occur 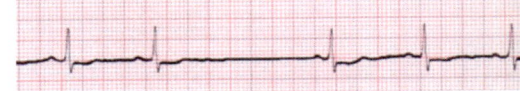
- **1° AV block-** prolonged PR interval (>.2 seconds) with no missed beats 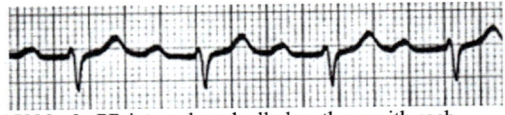
- **2° type 1 AV block-** PR interval gradually lengthens with each cycle until the last P wave in the series does not produce a QRS 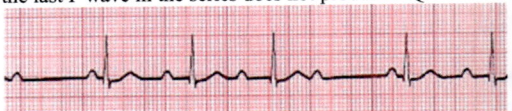
- **2° type 2 AV block-** Some P waves do not produce a QRS response (**treatment**: pacemaker) 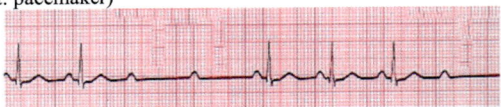
- **3° AV block (complete heart block)-** P waves and QRS have no correlation, if QRS is narrow and ventricular rate is 40-60 then it's a junctional focus, if QRS widened and rate is 20-40 then it's a ventricular focus (**treatment**: pacemaker) 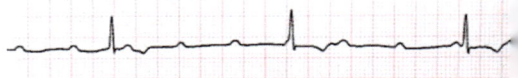
- **Right bundle branch block-** widened QRS with R,R' in V1/2 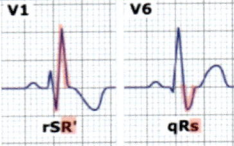
- **Left bundle branch block-** widened QRS with R,R' in V5/6

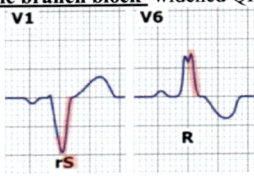

- o **Left anterior hemiblock-** prolonged or normal QRS duration with Q1S3 and left axis deviation
- o **Left posterior hemiblock-** prolonged or normal QRS duration with S1Q3 and right axis deviation

Axis:

- Is QRS positive or negative in leads I and AVF?

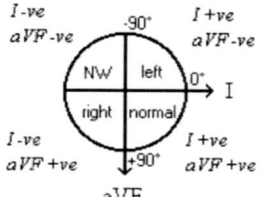

  o
  o Positive in I and AVF → normal axis
  o Positive in I and negative in AVF → left axis deviation
  o Negative in I and positive in AVF → right axis deviation
  o Negative in I and AVF → extreme right axis deviation

Hypertrophy:

- **Atrial hypertrophy:**
    o Look at lead V1 to look for a large, diphasic P wave, look at lead II for P wave morphology changes
    o **Right atrial hypertrophy-** V1 has a large, diphasic P wave with a tall initial component
    o **Left atrial hypertrophy-** V1 has a large, diphasic P wave with a wide terminal component

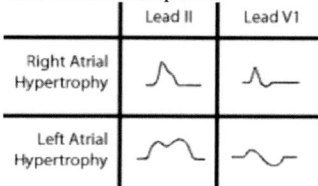

	Lead II	Lead V1
Right Atrial Hypertrophy		
Left Atrial Hypertrophy		

    o
- **Ventricular hypertrophy:**
    o Look at the R and S in leads V1, V5, V6, as well as right or left axis deviation
    o **Right ventricular hypertrophy-** R wave > S in V1 but R wave gets progressively smaller from V1-V6; S wave persists in V5/6; right axis deviation with slightly widened QRS

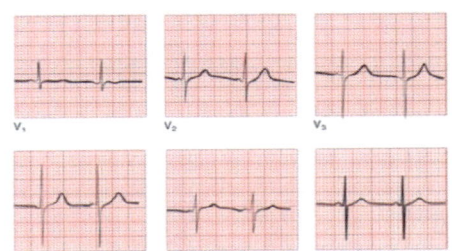

- **Left ventricular hypertrophy-** amplitude of S in V1 + amplitude of R in V5 is >35; left axis deviation with slightly widened QRS; inverted T wave slants downward gradually but up rapidly (not symmetrically)

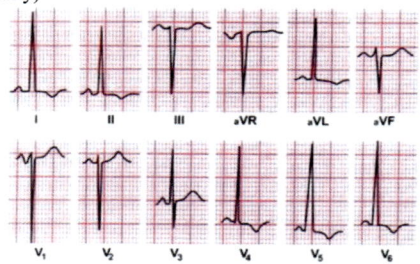

Infarction:

- Look for Q waves (necrosis)
- Look for ST depression or elevation (injury)
- Look for T wave inversion (ischemia)
- Look for changes in contiguous leads (know coronary anatomy)
- **Q waves:**
    - Necrosis of myocardial tissue
    - Significant Q waves are one mm wide, or 1/3 the amplitude (or more) of the QRS
    - Ignore lead AVR
    - Old infarct Q waves remain for a lifetime

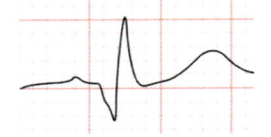

- **ST segment depression and elevation:**
    - Injury of myocardial tissue
    - ST elevation with significant Q waves indicates an acute or recent infarct
    - Returns to baseline with time

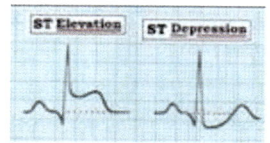

- **T wave inversion:**
    - Ischemia of myocardial tissue
    - Inverted T waves of ischemia are symmetric
    - Normally the T wave is upright when the QRS is upright, and inverted when the QRS is downward 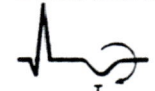
- **Look for changes in contiguous leads:**

Infarct location	Leads showing changes	Likely coronary artery involved
Inferior wall MI	II, III, aVF	RCA
Septal MI	V1-V2	LAD
Anterior wall MI	V3-V4	LAD
Anteroseptal wall MI	V1-V4	LAD
Lateral wall MI	I, aVL, V5-V6	Circumflex
Posterior wall MI	Prominent R in V1	RCA or circumflex
Right ventricular MI	ST elevation in V1 and right sided V4 with anterior wall MI	RCA

Approach to Arterial Blood Gases

- **Steps for ABG analysis:**
    - What is the pH? Acidemia or Alkalemia?
    - What is the primary disorder present? Metabolic or Respiratory?
    - Is there appropriate compensation?
    - Is the compensation acute or chronic?
    - Is there an anion gap?
    - If there is an anion gap, check the delta gap
    - What is the differential for the clinical presentation?
- **Normal values:**
    - pH: 7.35-7.45
    - pCO2: 35-45
    - HCO3-: 22-26
    - Anion gap: 10-14
    - Albumin: 4

What disorder is present?	pH	pCO2 or HCO3-
Respiratory acidosis	Low	High CO2
Metabolic acidosis	Low	Low HCO3-
Respiratory alkalosis	High	Low CO2
Metabolic alkalosis	High	High HCO3-

- **Is compensation acute or chronic?:**
    - Respiratory acidosis:
        - Acute- for every 10 increase in pCO2, HCO3- increases by 1 and pH decreases by 0.08
        - Chronic- for every 10 increase in pCO2, HCO3- increases by 4 and pH decreases by 0.03
    - Respiratory alkalosis:
        - Acute- for every 10 decrease in pCO2, HCO3- decreases by 2 and pH increases by 0.08
        - Chronic- for every 10 decrease in pCO2, HCO3- decreases by 5 and pH increases by 0.03
- **Winters formula:**
    - For metabolic acidosis, calculates the expected pCO2
    - pCO2= $1.5(HCO3-) + 8 \pm 2$
    - If serum pCO2 is greater than expected pCO2, an additional respiratory acidosis is present
- **Anion gap:**
    - AG = Na – (Cl + HCO3-)
    - Normal is 12 ± 2
    - Corrected anion gap for albumin = AG + 2.54(4-albumin)
- **Delta gap:**
    - Calculate if there is an anion gap present
    - Delta gap = (actual AG – 12) + HCO3-
    - If > 30 → additional metabolic alkalosis
    - If < 18 → additional non-gap metabolic acidosis
    - If 18-30 → no additional metabolic disorders

- **Anion gap metabolic acidosis differential (MUDPILERS):**
    - Methanol
    - Uremia
    - DKA, starvation ketoacidosis, EtOH ketoacidosis
    - Paraldehyde
    - INH, iron toxicity
    - Lactic acidosis
    - Ethylene glycol
    - Rhabdomyolysis
    - Salicyclates

- **Non anion gap metabolic acidosis differential (DURHAM):**
    - Diarrhea, ileostomy, colostomy, enteric fistula
    - Ureteral diversions or pancreatic fistulas
    - RTA type I or IV, early renal failure
    - Hyperalimentation, HCl administration
    - Acetazolamide, Addison's disease
    - Miscellaneous- post-hypocapnia, toluene, sevalemer, cholestyramine

- **Metabolic alkalosis differential:**
    - Calculate the urinary chloride to differentiate saline responsive vs. saline resistant
    - Must be off diuretics in order to interpret urine chloride

Saline responsive (urinary Cl <10)	Saline-resistant (urinary Cl >10)
Vomiting	If hypertensive: Cushings, Conn's, RAS, renal failure with alkali administration
NG suction	If not hypertensive: severe hypokalemia, hypomagnesia, Barterr's, Gittelman's, licorice ingestion
Over-diuresis	Exogenous corticosteroid administration
Post hypercapnia	

- **Respiratory alkalosis differential:**
    - Anxiety, pain, fever
    - Hypoxia, CHF
    - Lung disease with/without hypoxia- PE, reactive airway, PNA
    - CNS diseases
    - Drug use- salicylates, catecholamines, progesterone
    - Pregnancy
    - Sepsis, hypotension
    - Hepatic encephalopathy, liver failure
    - Mechanical ventilation
    - Hypothyroidism
    - High altitude

- **Respiratory acidosis differential:**
    - CNS depression- sedatives, narcotics, CVA
    - Neuromuscular disorders- acute or chronic
    - Acute airway obstruction- foreign body, tumor, reactive airway
    - Severe PNA, pulmonary edema, pleural effusion
    - Chest cavity problems- hemothorax, pneumothorax, flail chest
    - Chronic lung disease- obstructive or restrictive
    - Central hypoventilation, OSA

Electrolyte Repletion

- **Hypokalemia:**
    - Keep K > 4.0
    - 10 meq KCl PO/IV increases serum K by 0.1
    - IV KCl burns the veins, give with lidocaine
    - Oral KCl powder tastes bad, can give with orange juice (also has K), shorter acting
    - Oral KCl pill, hard to swallow
    - **Replete Mg first**, or the potassium won't stick
- **Hyperkalemia:**
    - For K > 5.0, if you think it's a trend, consider Kayexelate 15-30 g PO X 1, may repeat X 1 if no bowel movement in 4 hours
    - For **K > 6.0**, call the lab and make sure it wasn't hemolyzed. If it's real:
        - Check EKG
            - If EKG changes are present, give calcium gluconate 500-800 mg IV Q10 min prn
        - Temporizing measures:
            - D50 1 amp IV X 1 and Insulin 10 U IV X 1

- Calcium gluconate 1 amp IV (cardioprotective)
- NOT Kayexelate (with sorbitol in it) for acute
- Recheck the K, can give Lasix, may need dialysis if severe

- **Magnesium:**
    - Keep Mg > 2.0 (higher levels may decrease arrhythmias and improve mortality after MI, but the data are poor and/or contradictory)
    - Repletion:
        - MgSO4 4 g IV X 1 (for Mg <1.4)
        - MgSO4 6-8 g IV X 1 (for Mg <1.0)
        - MgOxide (400 mg PO BID) is good for patients with chronically low Mg

- **Calcium:**
    - Keep Ca > 8.5 or ionized Ca > 1.0
    - Corrected calcium = serum calcium – 0.8 X (normal albumin – serum albumin)
    - Treatment:
        - Calcium gluconate 1 amp IV (1 g = 4.5 meq Ca) and check a repeat ionized calcium)
        - If it is not an emergency, try calcium carbonate 1300 mg PO BID

- **Phosphate:**
    - Keep PO4 > 3.4
    - PO4 2.0-2.5 → 10-15 mmol Na-PO4 or K-PO4 IV X 1, OR 250 mg Neutraphos PO Q8 X 3
    - PO4 1.0-1.9 → 15-20 mmol Na-PO4 or K-PO4 IV X 1, OR 250 mg Neutrophos PO Q6 X 4
    - ≤1.0 → 20-25 mmol Na-PO4 or K-PO4 IV

Basic ICU Topics

Shock Differential

- **Distributive shock:**
    - **Septic shock:**
        - Caused by infection from bacteria, fungal, viral, parasites
    - **Non-septic:**
        - Inflammatory shock:
            - Burns, trauma, pancreatitis, post MI, post CABG, post cardiac arrest, viscus perforation, amniotic fluid embolism, fat embolism, idiopathic capillary leak syndrome
        - Neurogenic shock:
            - TBI, spinal cord injury (quadriparesis with bradycardia or paraplegia with tachycardia), neuro-axial anesthesia
        - Anaphylactic shock:
            - IgE-mediated (foods, meds, insect bites or stings), IgE-independent (iron dextran), nonimmunologic (exercise or heat-induced), idiopathic
        - Other:
            - Liver failure, transfusion reactions, vasoplegia (eg vasodilatory agents, cardiopulmonary bypass), toxic shock syndrome, toxicologic (heavy metals), beriberi
- **Cardiogenic shock:**
    - **Cardiomyopathic:**
        - MI (involving >40% of LV or extensive ischemia), severe RV infarction, acute exacerbation of severe heart failure from dilated cardiomyopathy, stunned myocardium from prolonged ischemia (cardiac arrest, hypotension, bypass), advanced septic shock, myocarditis, myocardial contusion, drug-induced (beta blockers)
    - **Arrhythmogenic:**
        - Tachycarrhythmia from atrial fibrillation/flutter, reentrant tachycardia), VT or VF
        - Bradyarrhythmia from complete heart block, 2nd degree type II AV block
    - **Mechanical:**
        - Severe valvular insufficiency, acute valvular rupture (papillary or chordae tendinae rupture, valvular abscess), critical valvular stenosis, acute or severe ventricular septal wall defect, ruptured ventricular wall aneurysm, atrial myxoma
- **Hypovolemic:**
    - **Hemorrhagic:**

- Trauma, GI bleeding (varices, peptic ulcer), intraoperative and postoperative bleeding, retroperitoneal bleeding (ruptured aortic aneurysm), aortic-enteric fistula, hemorrhagic pancreatitis, iatrogenic (inadvertent biopsy of arteriovenous malformation, or left ventricle), tumor or abscess erosion into major vessels, ruptured ectopic pregnancy, postpartum hemorrhage, uterine or vaginal hemorrhage (infection, tumors, lacerations), spontaneous peritoneal hemorrhage from bleeding diathesis
    - **Non-hemorrhagic:**
        - GI losses (diarrhea, vomiting, external drainage), skin losses (heat stroke, burns, dermatologic conditions), renal losses (excessive drug induced or osmotic diuresis, salt wasting nephropathies), hypoaldosternosim), third space losses into the extravascular space or body cavities (postoperative and trauma, intestinal obstruction, crush injury, pancreatitis, cirrhosis)
- **Obstructive:**
    - **Pulmonary vascular:**
        - Hemodynamically significant PE, severe pulmonary HTN, severe or acute obstruction of the pulmonic or tricuspid valve, venous air embolus
    - **Mechanical:**
        - Tension pneumothorax or hemothorax (trauma, iatrogenic), pericardial tamponade, constrictive pericarditis, restrictive cardiomyopathy, severe dynamic hyperinflation (elevated intrinsic PEEP), left or right ventricular outflow tract obstruction, abdominal compartment syndrome, aorto-caval compression (eg positioning, surgical retraction)
- **Mixed/unknown:**
    - **Endocrine:**
        - Adrenal insufficiency, thyrotoxicosis, myxedema coma
    - **Metabolic:**
        - Acidosis, hypothermia
    - **Other:**
        - Polytrauma with more than one shock category, acute shock etiology with pre-existing cardiac disease, late under-resuscitated shock, miscellaneous poisonings

Diagnosis	CVP	CO	PA	PCWP	SVR
Distributive	↓	↑↑	↓	↓	↓↓
Cardiogenic	↑	↓↓	↑	↑	↑↑
Hypovolemic	↓	↓-↑	↓	↓	↑↑
Obstructive	↑	↓~	↑↑	↓~	↑↑
Cardiac Tamponade	↑	↓	↑	↑	↑↑

Vasopressors

- Treat reversible causes of shock first, or ongoing treatment with vasopressors if the cause does not resolve with initial treatment
- Start vasopressors in shock if the patient is hypotensive with end organ dysfunction despite adequate fluid resuscitation (see sepsis spectrum)

Drug	Mechanism	Adverse effects	Notes
Levophed (NE)	α_1- ↑↑↑ β_1- ↑↑	Some arrhythmias, digital ischemia	First line in septic shock, other refractory shock
Vasopressin	Vasopressin receptor	Splanchanic, mesenteric, and digital ischemia	Synergistic with levophed in septic shock
Epinephrine	α_1- ↑↑↑↑↑ β_1- ↑↑↑↑↑	Significant tachycardia, ischemia	Anaphylactic shock first line, really potent
Phenylephrine	α_1- ↑↑↑	Causes relative bradycardia, don't use in cardiogenic shock	First line in left ventricular outflow tract obstruction with shock (aortic stenosis, HOCM)
Dopamine	Low dose- DA > β_1 Med dose- $\beta_1 > \beta_2$ High dose- $\alpha_1 > \beta_1$	Arrhythmias, ischemia	Low dose for renal failure (no evidence for this though), medium dose for cardiogenic, high septic
Dobutamine (inotrope)	β_1/β_2	Arrhythmias, ischemia	Used for cardiogenic shock

- Levophed still tends to be better for cardiogenic shock compared to dobutamine, which causes more arrhythmias and has the same mortality benefit
    - **SOAP II trial (2010, NEJM)-** In the treatment of shock, norepinephrine and dopamine compare similarly with respect to 28-day mortality, but dopamine is associated with an increased risk of arrhythmia

Indications for Intubation and Ventilatory Weaning

Indications for intubation:

- Clinical judgement is always important in the decision to intubate
- **General rules:**
    - Ventilator therapy indications:
        - Progressive hypoxemia
        - Progressive hypercapnia

- Neurologic deterioration
- Respiratory muscle failure
  - Sustained tachypnea (RR $\geq$ 30/min) is frequently a sign of impending respiratory failure
- Three questions can help with the decision to intubate or not:
  - **Is there failure of airway maintenance or protection?**
    - If the patient is not able to phonate or swallow secretions, this is a sign they need to be intubated
    - If they are altered to the point where they cannot maintain their away then they need to be intubated
  - **Is there failure of oxygenation or ventilation?**
    - The inability to oxygenate despite supplemental oxygen poses an immediate life threat and, with rare exceptions, mandates intubation
    - Trial of noninvasive positive pressure ventilation if tolerated
    - Pulse oximetry provides an accurate estimate of arterial oxygen tension, but can be unreliable when peripheral perfusion is compromised
    - ABGs should be interpreted judiciously, for example, an "unimpressive" ABG in a severe asthmatic may postpone intubation as the PCO2 begins to increase, but this can be from respiratory muscle fatigue and they need to be intubated
    - CO2 levels can be used, and are especially good if elevated if the person is altered, however, chronic CO2 retainers (COPD pts) can have elevated PCO2 levels normally, and should be tried on BiPap first
  - **Is there an anticipated need for intubation?**
    - Patients that are getting worse clinically but are still protecting their airway, oxygenating and ventilating well, still may need eventual intubation
    - If the patient is being transferred to radiology for imaging, or to another facility, it is better to secure the airway preemptively than to face an emergency unplanned airway

[Flowchart:
- Is there failure of airway maintenance or protection?
  - Yes → Intubate
  - No → Is there failure of oxygenation or ventilation?
    - Yes → NIPPV candidate?
      - No → Intubate
      - Yes → Success?
        - No → Intubate
        - Yes → Observe
    - No → Does the anticipated clinical Course require intubation?
      - No → Observe
      - Yes → Intubate]

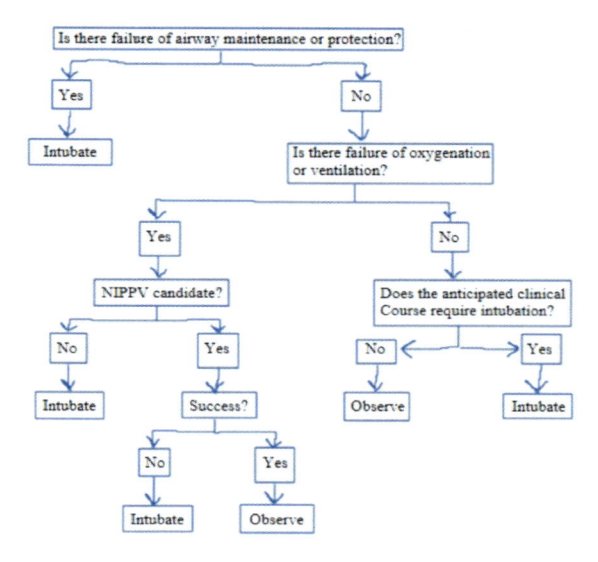

Ventilator Weaning:

- **Daily** assessment whether the patient should undergo a spontaneous breathing trial should be performed
    - Assessment includes:
        - Reason why they were intubated is controlled
        - No significant electrolyte abnormalities
        - Vital signs stable (generally off of pressors, HR <140)
        - Minimal secretions
        - Adequate cough
        - PaO2/FiO2 >200 with FiO2 <50%
        - No myocardial ischemia
        - PaCO2 normal or back to their baseline
        - PEEP ≤ 5
        - Arousable, generally GCS ≥ ~8, opens eyes and without agitation
        - Inspiratory effort present
- **Daily** sedation holidays
    - **Efficacy and safety of a paired sedation and ventilator weaning protocol for mechanically ventilated patients in intensive care (Awakening and Breathing Controlled trial) (2008, The Lancet)-** A wake up and breathe protocol that pairs daily spontaneous awakening trials (ie, interruption of sedatives) with daily spontaneous breathing trials results in better outcomes for mechanically ventilated patients in intensive care
- **Weaning protocol:**
    - Respiratory therapist does this protocol
    - Place patient on pressure support (CPAP or T piece) for at least 30 minutes (30-120 minutes)
    - Rapid shallow breathing index measured
        - RR/(TV/100)- value >105 predicts failure

- If failure is due to tachypnea, you should assess if this tachypnea was accompanied by low or high tidal volumes
    - If high tidal volumes, then the tachypnea was most likely from anxiety, and you can try benzos or opiates to relieve the anxiety and try again
    - If low tidal volumes, this is most likely from respiratory failure and should not try to extubate
  - Cuff leak test
    - Tests for laryngeal edema
    - If positive, this means there is not laryngeal edema significant enough to prevent air passage out of the respiratory tract to the mouth
    - If it is negative, give methylprednisolone 20mg IV Q4h starting 12h pre-extubation (decreases edema and gives a 50% reduction in re-intubation) (Lancet 2007;369:1003)
  - Negative inspiratory force (NIF) test
    - Measures diaphragm muscle strength
    - If the value is ≤ -20, this is a good predictor of extubation success (the more negative the value the better)
- If the above parameters are not met, then you need to think of why they failed and what you are going to do about it
- If all the parameters are met, extubate the patient
  - If the patient has COPD or is a chronic CO2 retainer, you can extubate them to BiPap
  - For most patients, you can extubate them to nasal cannula
- Approximately 15% of patients fail extubation
  - In these patients, you should not try noninvasive positive pressure oxygen therapy, they should be re-intubated

DKA Initial Labs and Management

- **Initial labs typically seen in DKA:**
  - Glucose 300-800
  - Increased ketones
  - HCO3- 0-15
  - pH 6.8-7.3
  - Na can be decreased, normal, or increased
  - K can be decreased, normal, or increased (total body K is usually depleted however despite the initial value)
  - Phosphorus can be normal to increased
  - Cr and BUN usually increased
  - WBC count usually increased
  - Amylase usually increased
  - Hemoglobin and hematocrit usually increased (from dilution)
  - LDH normal to increased
- **Fluids:**
  - NS 1-2 L bolus initially, then:
    - 1 L/hr for 4 hrs, then

- 250-500 ml/hr for 4 hrs, then
- 100-250 ml/hr
- Give ½ NS if corrected Na is >145
- Change to D5 NS 200 mg/hr when blood glucose <250

- **Insulin:**
  - Initial long acting insulin (usually given in ED) with insulin drip started
  - Check blood glucose every hour
  - BMP Q4h to check anion gap and K+
  - If current blood glucose >250 AND:
    - Has not decreased by >20 → increase the rate of insulin drip by 50%
    - Has not decreased by >20 but blood glucose <200 → no change
    - Has decreased by >20 → decreased rate of insulin drip by 50%
    - **This is done by the nurse in the DKA order set**
  - Overlap IV insulin with subQ insulin (calculated by weight based) when anion gap has closed twice for 2 hours, then allow patient to eat

- **Potassium replacement:**
  - Replace once K level is <5

Common Medications

Cardiac Medications:

Heart Failure:

Medication	Dose
Metoprolol Succinate	Start 12.5 mg, max 200 mg — Once a day
Metoprolol Tartrate	Start 25 mg, max 100 mg — Twice a day
Carvedilol	Start 3.125 mg, max 25 mg — Twice a day
Lisinopril	Start 5 mg, max 40 mg — Once a day
Valsartan	Start 40 mg, max 320 mg — Once a day
Furosemide	Start 20 mg, max 80 (sort of) — Twice a day
Spironolactone	25 mg — Once a day
BiDil (hydralazine/isosorbide dinitrate)	37.5/25 mg — Three times a day

Max out the beta blocker and ACEI/ARB before adding Spironolactone or BiDil. Both spironolactone and BiDil have one dose. Do not titrate Spironolactone and BiDil up in heart failure like the others.

Coronary Artery Disease:

Medication	Dose
Metoprolol Succinate	Start 12.5 mg, max 200 mg — Once a day
Metoprolol Tartrate	Start 25 mg, max 100 mg — Twice a day
Carvedilol	Start 3.125 mg, max 25 mg — Twice a day
Lisinopril	Start 5 mg, max 40 mg — Once a day
Valsartan	Start 40 mg, max 320 mg — Once a day
Aspirin	81 or 325 mg — Once a day
Rosuvastatin	Low 10 mg, goal 40 mg — Once a day
Atorvastatin	Low 20 mg, goal 40-80 mg — Once a day
Clopidogrel	75 mg — Once a day

Everyone with coronary artery disease needs to be on Aspirin, a Statin, a beta blocker, and an ACEI/ARB. Other medications are used for anti-anginal properties or blood pressure control. Notice the similarities in medications for heart failure and coronary artery disease.

Hypertension:

Medication	Dose	Other Information
Hydrochlorothiazide	Start 25 mg	Causes hypokalemia/hypercalcemia
Lisinopril	40 mg	Causes hyperkalemia, angioedema, cough
Valsartan	320 mg	Causes hyperkalemia
Amlodipine	10 mg	Anti-anginal, most expensive cheap HTN med
Labetalol	200 mg TID	Only beta blocker for HTN, use in ESRD
Spironolactone	25 mg	Last ditch med, hyperkalemia
Clonidine	0.1-0.3 mg TID	Get patients off this, it's awful but works
Labetalol	10 mg IV	If sys BP >180 and HR >90
Hydralazine	10 mg IV	If sys BP >180 and HR <90

Hospital goal is <180/<110. Clinic goal is generally <140/<80, but, **see JNC-8 guidelines**

Respiratory Medications:

COPD:

Medication	Dose	Other Information
Albuterol	90 mcg	prn
Tiotropium	18 mcg	Spiriva, once a day
Budenoside/Formoterol	Disk, puff twice daily	Pulmicort BID, NOT for hosp
Fluticasone/Salmeterol	Disk, puff twice daily	Advair BID. NOT for hosp
Prednisone	40 mg	PO
Albuterol/Ipratropium	2.5/0.5 mg	Duoneb, Q4h prn SOB, for hosp
Methylprednisolone	125 mg IV	Solumedrol
Doxycycline or Azithromycin	100 mg PO BID or 500 mg PO	For azithro, 250 mg PO after 1st day

Recognize that the same medications used for outpatient are used for inpatient, for the most part. Advair and Pulmicort are typically not used for exacerbations. You replace them with methylprednisolone, which gives them in patient criteria. Then rapidly adjust to prednisone after they meet inpatient criteria. DPE-4 inhibitors are also used for COPD. Use uptodate to know them if you really need them.

Asthma:

Medication	Dose	Other Information
Albuterol	90 mcg	Prn
Budenoside/Formoterol	Disk, puff twice daily	Pulmicort BID, NOT for hosp
Fluticasone/Salmeterol	Disk, puff twice daily	Advair BID. NOT for hosp
Prednisone	40 mg	PO
Albuterol/Ipratropium	2.5/0.5 mg	Duoneb, Q4h prn SOB, for hosp
Methylprednisolone	125 mg IV	Solumedrol
Magnesium	2 g IV	Last resort
SubQ epinephrine	0.1 mg SubQ	Last resort

Notice the similarities between COPD and asthma; they are essentially the same. Leukotriene antagonists work essentially like inhaled corticosteroids, and are added to asthma but not to COPD.

Gastrointestinal Medications:

Constipation:

Medication	Dose	Other Information
Colace/Docusate	100 mg BID	Stool softener, opiate ppx
Senna	8.6 mg BID, 17.2 mg BID	Motility agent, opiate ppx
Lactulose	20 mg/ 30 mL prn	Motility, acute constipation
GoLytely	1 gallon	They will defecate
Disimpaction		Best way to defecate and stimulate the bowel
Fleet, soap suds, tap water enema		Nurse driven, loosens stool, do after disimpaction attempt
Lactulose retention enema		Lactulose through a rectal tube into rectum (or foley), clamp it, let sit then open it up

Strength increases as you go down the list. Do Colace + Senna for opiate constipation prophylaxis. Whenever you give a motility agent also give a stool softener. Having a lot of contractility against a hard stool hurts. You should be the one to attempt disimpaction (the intern).

Emesis:

Medication	Dose	Other Information
Diphenhydramine	25 mg	When you think they do not have nausea, but want to give them something
Promethazine (Phenergan)	12.5 mg IV, 25 mg PO	Start here
Metoclopramide (Reglan)	10 mg IV	Use only in gastroparesis, avoid in gastric outlet obstruction, causes tardive dyskinesia
Ondansetron (Zofran)	4 mg IV, 8 mg PO	Strongest we have
Dexamethasone	8, 10, or 12 mg PO or IV	When nothing else works
Lorazepam (Ativan)	0.5 or 1 mg PO or IV	Adjunct, don't give this often

Strength increases as you go down the list (except lorazepam).

Antibiotics:

Organism	Gram stain features	Clinical importance
Enterococci	Gram + cocci in chains	UTI, endocarditis
Streptococci	Gram + cocci in chains	A: pharyngitis B: neonatal sepsis
Viridians streptococci	Gram + cocci in chains	Endocarditis, abscess, dental carries
Streptococcus pneumoniae	Gram + diplococci in chains	Community acquired PNA, septic shock, meningitis
Staph aureus	Gram + cocci in clusters	Cellulitis, abscess, septic shock, endocarditis
Coagulase negative staph	Gram + cocci in clusters	Bacteremia, infection of prosthetic devices
E. coli	Gram – rods	UTI, septic shock, hemorrhagic colitis
Klebsiella spp	Gram – rods	UTI, septic shock, PNA
Enterobacter/citrobacter	Gram – rods	UTI, PNA, septic shock
Pseudomonas aeruginosa	Gram – rods	UTI, PNA, septic shock
Neisseria meningitidis	Gram – diplococci	Septic shock, meningitis
Haemophilus influenzae	Gram – coccobacillus	Respiratory tract infections
Clostridium spp	Gram + rod, anaerobic	Tetanus, botulism, infections of soft tissue, abdominal sepsis, abscess
Peptococcus/peptostreptococcus spp	Gram + cocci in chains, anaerobic	Infections of soft tissue, abdominal sepsis, abscess
Bacteroides/prevotella spp	Gram – rod, anaerobic	Infections of soft tissue, abdominal sepsis, abscess

Empiric Treatment:

Diagnosis	Empiric Antibiotics	Duration
CAP	Ceftriaxone and azithromycin	5-7 days
HAP	Vancomycin and Zosyn	5-7 days
UTI	Ceftriaxone (inpt) or Cipro (outpt pyelo), or Nitrofurantoin (outpt cystitis)	3 days for uncomplicated 7 days for complicated 10 days for pyelo 14 days for abscess
Meningitis	Vancomycin and ceftriaxone and dexamethasone ± ampicillin (immunocompromised)	7 days
Cellulitis	MRSA- vanc, clinda, bactrim Strep- Keflex, clinda, augmentin	7 days
Diabetic foot	Vancomycin and zosyn	
Diverticulitis	Cipro and metronidazole or zosyn	5-7 days
Cholangitis	Cipro and metronidazole or zosyn	5-7 days

Medication	Dose	Route	Timing
Vancomycin	1 g	IV	Q12h
Zosyn	3.375 g	IV	Q6h
Zosyn	4.5 g	IV	Q8h
Zosyn	2.225 g	IV	Q8h
Cipro	400 mg	IV	Q12h
Cipro	500 mg	PO	Q12h
Ceftriaxone	1 g	IV	Daily
Ceftriaxone	2 g	IV	Daily
Metronidazole	500 mg	IV	Q8h
Clindamycin	500 mg	IV	Q8h
Azithromycin	500 mg	IV	Daily
Moxifloxacin	500 mg	IV	Daily
Nafcillin	1 g	IV	Q4h

- Collect cultures before starting antibiotics
- Many antibiotics require renal dosing, such as vancomycin, if you are unsure, call the pharmacist or do dosing per pharmacy
- ID approval is required for many antibiotics depending on the hospital. Call ID fellow for approval when required.
- Use Sanford guide and hospital antibiograms to help
- **Factors to consider when choosing antibiotics:**
    - Patients recent antibiotic use
    - Hospital flora
    - Presence of underlying disease
    - Available culture data- current and past
    - Risk for drug resistant pathogens
        - Antibiotics within the last 90 days
        - Hospitalization for ≥ 5 days

- Antibiotic resistance in the community
- Immunosuppressive disease and/or therapy
- Presence of risk factors for resistance
  - Location:
    - Where did the patient become ill? Travel? Exposure?
    - Where did the infection originate anatomically?
    - Where in the body has/will the infection spread to?
  - What bug are you treating?

- **Beta lactams:**
  - Penicillin- pneumococcus, strep, enterococcus, N. meningitidis, syphilis, listeria, leptospirosis, and oral anaerobes
  - Amoxicillin- same as penicillin with expanded activity against gram negatives (E. coli, proteus, H. influenza, H. pylori, N meningitidis, shigella, klebsiella), covers most spirochetes (lyme).
  - Oxacillin/nafcillin/dicloxacillin- only for staph (except MRSA), pneumococcus, and other strep
  - Piperacillin and Ticarcillin- piperacillin covers pseudomonas, strep, enterococcus, does not cover MRSA

- **Cephalosporins:**
  - 1st generation:
    - Cefazolin- staph, non enterococcal strep, prophylactic in clean surgeries, cellulitis, folliculitis. Limited in respiratory tract infections, animal bites, or surgeries involving colon
  - 2nd generation:
    - Cefuroxime- respiratory infections- strep pneumoniae, H. infleunzae, and Moraxella, meningitis due to pneumococcus, H. flu, and N. meningitidis. Limited with enteric organisms/abdominal anaerobes
    - Cefoxitin/Cefotetan- intrabominal infections especially anaerobes. Limited by staph and other gram positives.
  - 3rd generation:
    - Cefotaxime and ceftriaxone- good for staph, and non-enterococcal strep, broad coverage of gram negative and oral anaerobes, CNS, pulmonary, endovascular, GI infections, excluding gut anaerobes), sinusitis, otitis, head and neck. Limited by no pseudomonas coverage, ceftriaxone can cause biliary sludging and limits its utility in treating biliary tree infections
    - Ceftazidime- good for gram negative coverage including pseudomonas, febrile neutropenia, CNS infections,- good for pseudomonas meningitis. Limited by reduced activity against gram positives and oral anaerobes.
  - 4th generation:
    - Cefepime and cepirome- Enterobacter, citrobacter, and serratia, pseudomonas, gram positives, use din neutropenic fever and CNS infections

- **Carbapenems:**
  - Imipenem- more activity against gram positive bacteria than meropenem or ertapenem
  - Ertapenem- good for aerobic gram negatives, **poor for pseudomonas**
  - Meropenem- good for aerobic gram negatives
  - Doripenem- good for CNS coverage and pseudomonas

- **Fluoroquinolones:**
    o Ciprofloxacin- covers most aerobic gram negatives including pseudomonas, penetrates CNS, prostate, lungs, limited against staph
    o Non-ciprofloxacin quinolones (oxafloxacin, levofloxacin, moxifloxacin, gemifloxacin)- great for respiratory pathogens, only levofloxacin covers pseudomonas, covers some atypicals- mycoplasma, chlamydia, legionella.
    o **Can prolong QT interval**, tendon rupture, CNS toxicity
    o **Commonly causes C. diff**
- **Macrolides:**
    o Erythromycin, clarithromycin, azithromycin- broad spectrum against gram positives including strep, staph (MSSA). Good for atypical organism such as mycoplasma, chlamydia, legionella. Covers N. gonorrhea, H. flu, legionella
    o Caution that can cause QT prolongation
- **Clindamycin:**
    o Reasonable gram positive aerobic coverage against strep and many staph including MRSA. Special role in treating strep in necrotizing fasciitis
    o Anaerobic coverage better than penicillin but worse than metronidazole
    o **Commonly causes C. diff**
- **Metronidazole:**
    o No aerobic activity
    o Does not stand alone for mixed infections
    o Good for anaerobes
    o C. diff, parasites, bacterial vaginosis
    o May require reduced dose in liver disease
    o Can increase effect of warfarin
- **Pseudomonas covering antibiotics:**
    o Zosyn, aminoglycosides, cephalosporins (ceftazidime, cefepime), fluoroquinolones (ciprofloxacin, levofloxacin), carbapenems (imipenem, meropenem), aztreonam, colistin
- **Anaerobe covering antibiotics:**
    o Flagyl, clindamycin, zosyn, unasyn, augmentin, carbapenem, moxifloxacin, tigecycline
- **MRSA covering antibiotics:**
    o Bactrim, clindamycin, doxycycline, vancomycin, linezolid, tigecycline, daptomycin (do not use in lungs)
- **VRE covering antibiotics:**
    o Linezolid, tigecycline, daptomycin

Notes

Notes

Notes

Notes

Made in the USA
Middletown, DE
30 April 2022